Principles and Practice Series

NON-INVASIVE CARDIOVASCULAR MONITORING

Principles and Practice Series

NON-INVASIVE CARDIOVASCULAR MONITORING

BERNARD HAYES

Former Consultant Anaesthetist, City Hospital, Birmingham

Series Editors

C E W HAHN

University Lecturer in Anaesthetics,
University of Oxford,
and
Consultant in Clinical Measurement,
Oxford Radcliffe Hospital

and

A P ADAMS

Professor of Anaesthetics,
University of London,
United Medical and Dental Schools of
Guy's and St Thomas's Hospitals
and
Honorary Consultant Anaesthetist,
Guy's, King's and St Thomas' Hospitals, London

First published in 1997
by the BMJ Publishing Group, BMA House, Tavistock Square,
London WC1H 9JR

British Library Cataloguing in Publication Data

A catalogue record for this book is available from the British Library

ISBN 0-7279-1038-8

Typeset, printed and bound in Great Britain by
Latimer Trend & Company Ltd., Plymouth

Contents

Note: A separate alphabetical referencing system has been used for the figure sources. The figure reference list is on p. 222.

Preface

The editors of the *Principles and Practice* series identified a need for a coherent practical overview of non-invasive cardiovascular monitoring, as opposed to a purely academic treatment of the subject, and they approached me to be the author. As a user of many of the techniques of non-invasive cardiovascular monitoring, I was aware that there was no volume drawing together the principal non-invasive methods, and thought that I might be reasonably placed to give a broadly based practical insight into the techniques, their basis and their application. It was in this spirit that I undertook the task.

The book takes into account the historical development of the techniques where this has a bearing on the nature of the devices used, the manner of their adoption and their more recent exploitation. It is directed at those who need to have a grasp of the essential principles and of the pros and cons of this type of monitoring in the day-to-day activities of various fields of medical and related endeavour. Thus, I have had in mind: those who use the techniques intensively during their training, as is the case for anaesthetists and those working in accident and emergency teams; nurses, especially those who take part in routine monitoring of this kind, as in critical care areas and in anaesthetic and recovery nursing; and also those who may now be spurred on to using non-invasive cardiovascular monitoring more extensively outside the acute hospital in general practice and the community and in the home. I have therefore tried to stress the practical aspects because there are many more detailed texts dealing with each of the groups of techniques in a more rigorous fashion.

The monitoring of expired carbon dioxide, as in capnometry, has been omitted deliberately because it is strictly speaking a respiratory approach which provides information about the cardiovascular system only inferentially and has, in any case, been covered in a companion volume in this series. Similarly, pulse oximetry has been dealt with thoroughly in another companion volume.

Medical alarms have been the source of confusion and irritation on account of their obvious shortcomings, especially where they are numerous, as in critical care areas and the operating suite. Recent developments give some immediate advantages in the current clinical setting and the promise of better things to come. The coverage here, although valid for non-invasive cardiovascular monitoring, is therefore directed at the general philosophy of alarms and their wider clinical application. I hope that this section will bring some understanding to users who work with alarms in difficult circumstances.

Bernard Hayes

1 Introduction

General

Monitoring is a term open to a variety of interpretations. Derived from the ancient Greek μονεω (pronounced "moneo"), meaning "I warn", it is used today more loosely to describe the transfer of information or data. Thus, monitoring may refer to the acquisition of data, its retention and its processing, as well as the provocation of alarms. Outside the field of medicine and related disciplines, we may speak of monitoring in relation to the supervision of, for example, electricity and gas distribution systems and of the plants generating the electricity or gas. It may equally be applied to epidemiological gathering of data with a view to possible action. At a more fundamental level it may be applied, perhaps incorrectly, to the simple recording of data, especially by automated instruments, as in data logging. For the purposes of this volume, a mixture of these usages has been adopted, the level of "monitoring" being generally clear from the context.

"Non-invasive" is a term now accepted as implying that the method does not breach the integrity of either external or internal body surfaces. Measurement of physiological values is thus dependent on the sensing of related phenomena at convenient sites on the surface of the body. It is debatable as to what extent these surfaces must be external or whether, for practical purposes, some degree of intrusion into orifices and cavities may be legitimately referred to as non-invasive. For example, the introduction of an auriscope would probably not be thought of as invasive. It is thus convenient to include procedures which do not breach a surface and which do not occasion discomfort as a result of their partial introduction into easily accessible orifices.

This volume is concerned with non-invasive cardiovascular monitoring, implying the use of devices which obtain information (or values) from the body without transgressing skin or mucous membranes or entering inner body cavities. The term "indirect" is also sometimes used, in contradistinction to the term "direct", often applied to invasive cardiovascular monitoring, especially that of blood pressure. Direct invasive blood pressure monitoring provides a good example of the distinction, in that a blood vessel is cannulated and the pressure information drawn directly from the activity inside the blood vessel, whereas the indirect non-invasive approach requires that the pressure be inferred from the pressure

1

generated in an externally applied device where the behaviour can be correlated with that of the interior of the blood vessel.

Pulse oximetry, although extremely valuable as a non-invasive monitoring tool, is not dealt with here, as it is comprehensively covered in another companion volume in this series.[1]

Merits of the non-invasive approach

It may be asked what merit there is in using inferential methods when direct techniques are available. The most obvious answer lies in the breaching of bodily integrity intrinsic to invasive methods referred to above, with the consequent possibility of tissue damage and sepsis. More pertinent is the degree of correlation which can be achieved when indirect non-invasive methods are applied. This varies with the nature of the application, the circumstances of measurement and the uses to which the resultant data will be put. Some non-invasive methods have been available for many years and individual techniques, e.g. sphygmomanometry, have stood the test of time.

Moreover, invasive measurements are necessarily cause for concern to conscious subjects and, whilst they may be made readily acceptable by, for example, local anaesthesia and appropriate reassurance, there have been strong pressures for the substitution of non-invasive methods when these are appropriate. Not least among such pressures has been the emergence of an increasing threat of litigation in association with what may be regarded by individuals and the general public as invasions of their personal domain of privacy, especially when complications occur.

In a most thought-provoking paper, Pask[2] foresaw the increasing use of automatic monitoring devices and yet wondered whether the correct variables were being monitored automatically. He feared that instrumentation might be used simply to automate the acquisition of information formerly elicited by an astute clinical observer, and that the available technology might not be used to measure possibly more useful variables not necessarily amenable to being elicited clinically. Much of the cardiovascular monitoring used today still exploits time-honoured principles but, fortunately, more recent methods have come on the diagnostic and therapeutic scene as the result of advances in specific materials and measurement technologies. In particular, there has been a sharp movement from invasive to non-invasive methods where the safety of the patients permits it and reduced morbidity and greater patient comfort demand it.

Historical outline

General

Monitoring probably has its origins in what would now be called clinical investigation, the dominant driving force being the desire to obtain new information about human physiology and its disorders. In past decades, when the pursuit of knowledge perhaps transcended other aspects of the human condition, it was considered perfectly reasonable to subject individuals to uncomfortable, even painful, procedures provided the extant criteria for the expansion of knowledge were satisfied.

Epidemiological studies prompted the development of methods of data gathering which could be used confidently in the field. Methods which could be used by relative non-experts proved particularly attractive. The epidemiological study of hypertension has eloquently demonstrated the value of the simple, rugged sphygmomanometer as just such an instrument. The extension of the principle into the out-patient clinic, the general practice surgery, the health clinic, and mobile screening units has brought with it the demand for similar rugged, reliable, non-invasive instruments which can be used by health professionals from diverse backgrounds and also by patients and other lay persons to produce results comparable with those previously obtained only by invasive methods.

Invasive methods have, until quite recently, been dominant in critical care and seem likely to remain so for the foreseeable future. Nevertheless, non-invasive techniques offer sufficient promise in a number of applications, not least cardiovascular, to prompt their use in certain circumstances.

Specific developments

In the field of cardiovascular monitoring, the electrocardiogram (ECG), pulse and blood pressure monitoring, and means of estimating cardiac performance are the most obvious examples of non-invasive monitoring to have achieved success.

Clinical considerations

Application

Some general principles may be stated concerning the clinical application of non-invasive cardiovascular monitoring. The variable and its parameters must be genuinely conveniently accessible to the non-invasive approach

3

and must produce results where accuracy and repeatability are consistent with the clinical objective. This has implications that may not be immediately obvious to those accustomed to using invasive measurement techniques in a particular aspect of their work. For example, the method used may produce output in a form which becomes familiar or habitual. That output may give rise to derived information that, whilst of value, may or may not be essential to clinical management. The technical requirements of the method may place restrictions on data production in terms of high accuracy and modes of display that, again, are commonly accepted for those techniques, but that may exceed the basic requirements of the health professional concerned in his or her particular clinical setting. Therefore, the possibility of using non-invasive methods should be viewed against criteria appropriate to:

- the tasks for which it is envisaged the device will be used;
- the level of information required;
- the manner of presentation acceptable to the user;
- compatibility with other equipment to which it might be connected.

In summary, the user should determine what the real needs are, rather than simply whether the non-invasive method performs in the same way as the more familiar invasive instrument.

Medico-legal aspects

Although it is impossible to prejudge the outcome of medico-legal actions launched in respect of the use of medical devices and associated methods, it is useful to reflect on the causes of such legal actions and the means of reducing the likelihood of their being contemplated.

Cardiovascular monitoring, like other forms of monitoring, is a relatively recent development which marries the concepts of convenience of repetitive measurement with the notion of surveillance. Making repeated measurements with a plethora of instruments does not of itself confer greater safety, but must be combined with vigilance on the part of the person responsible for the measurements in relation to taking a mental note of the results of the measurements, recording them and subsequently acting upon them. As Aitkenhead has pointed out: "It is now almost impossible to defend a claim in which appropriate monitoring has not been used during anaesthesia if the injury might have been prevented by earlier diagnosis of a physiological 'abnormality'".[3] It is assumed here that acting upon the results of measurements includes the decision *not* to take positive action, but merely to note and to continue to observe. This last is of importance, since it is popularly inferred that the display of a result or a

4

warning based upon it should prompt overt action. In fact, the judicious clinician may legitimately decide that no action is yet necessary.

To develop this theme, monitoring has come to be regarded by those inside and outside health care as a means of ensuring additional safety in its own right. As can be seen, this is only so if the user has received proper training on the device, its method of use and its application, and is cognisant of the appropriate responses to be made to the results of the measurements. Studies concerned with the transfer of critically ill patients between treatment sites tend to confirm this view[4,5]

Other factors have influenced the introduction of monitoring into certain environments and its extension, once it has become established in a particular area.[6] A good example is the advent of "minimal monitoring standards" in anaesthesia.[7] In response to pressure from medical indemnity organisations, a list of measurement functions has been prepared that can be applied to the practice of anaesthesia.[8] There is still much uncertainty as to whether all or any the measures described have contributed directly to the greater safety of patients.[9,10] However, adoption of such standards[11] serves to remind all anaesthetists of the potential hazards and the role of monitoring in helping to avoid them every time an anaesthetic is undertaken. Moreover, in the USA at least, medical insurance premiums have been limited as a result. The Association of Anaesthetists of Great Britain and Ireland has published its own guidance on monitoring during anaesthesia[12] and an International Task Force on Anaesthesia Safety has made recommendations[13] which, although not confined to monitoring, convey a similar message and have been adopted by the World Federation of Societies of Anaesthesiologists.

The recording of critical incidents encountered in medical practice might be expected to shed light on the part played by monitoring. The Australian Incident Monitoring Study[14] has made a significant contribution to our understanding, making the point that although human error may feature in mishaps, the prime cause of an incident or accident is often a system-based problem. This study stresses the importance of appreciating what particular monitoring techniques can offer and, hence, which monitors are worthy of selection. This is emphasised in a separate report from the same source.[15]

It is now well established that applying monitoring implies taking care[16] and that the absence of suitable cardiovascular monitoring in certain clinical circumstances might be construed as negligent practice. Another consideration is whether or not non-invasive (i.e. "indirect") monitoring could be seen as being less effective than invasive (or "direct") monitoring. It is important that non-invasive monitoring shows good correlation with invasive methods or, at least, that the information provided by it shows comparable clinical usefulness.

Cost implications

Non-invasive instruments are not necessarily less expensive than their invasive counterparts. Indeed, the need for different forms of artefact rejection makes such a comparison difficult. The costs of both types of instrument depend upon the application, the quality of the data expected, convenience, the ability to connect them with other devices and a number of other considerations, prominent among which is the training needed. What is certain is that an elaborate specification for the device does not necessarily imply that the more expensive (or elaborate) instrument is better for the task in hand. In Europe, the Medical Device Directives lay down important requirements which determine the design characteristics of the devices to some extent.[17] National, International (IEC/ISO) and European (CEN) Standards may be invoked by manufacturers and suppliers so that compliance with them implies a certain basic level of safety and/or performance. These will be referred to at appropriate points in the text. However, the selector of the apparatus must be satisfied that the specification is appropriate to the clinical application and must consider the various trade-offs such as desirable enhanced performance and features, presentation, user preference and the like.

General methodologies

Historical

Several non-invasive cardiovascular measurements have been available for over 100 years.

Blood pressure was originally measured non-invasively by an occluding cuff and a means of detecting pressure changes downstream of the cuff. This was first achieved by applying a finger to the pulse and reading the pressure in the cuff from a suitable pressure indicator. Later, the pulse was detected by virtue of the sound vibrations produced beyond the point of occlusion as the pressure was released or by mechanical means.

Recent

More recently, the onset of flow has been detected by the use of transmitted or reflected light, whilst pulsations have been detected by various transducers. Transducers are devices which convert one form of energy into another. Thus, the change in a transmitted light signal may be converted into an electrically equivalent signal which may, in turn, be amplified to provide a useful output. Pressure transducers may sense pressure within the occluding cuff or outside it.

The electrical impulses generated by the heart have long been known to represent its activity when detected as potential differences at certain points on the exterior of the chest.

Ultrasound has been used to detect the flow in blood vessels beyond an occluding cuff, the transducer in this instance consisting of both an emitter of ultrasound and a corresponding detector. More inferentially, ultrasound has been used to estimate the output of the heart or that of its ventricles. In some instances, as in the estimation of cardiac output, natural electrical potentials have been recorded from the surface of the body which can be correlated with changes in the cardiac output.

1 Moyle JBT. *Pulse oximetry*. London: BMJ Publishing Group, 1994.
2 Pask EA. Hunt the signal. *Proc Roy Soc Med* 1965; **58**: 757–66.
3 Aitkenhead AK. The pattern of litigation against anaesthetists. *Br J Anaesth* 1994; **73**: 10–21.
4 Reeve WG, Runcie CJ, Reidy J, Wallace PG. Current practice in transferring critically ill patients in the west of Scotland. *BMJ* 1990; **300**: 85–7.
5 Oakley PA. The need for standards for inter-hospital transfer. *Anaesthesia* 1994; **49**: 565–6.
6 Sykes MK. Essential monitoring. *Br J Anaesth*; 1987; **59**: 901–12.
7 Cass NM, Crosby WM, Holland RB. Minimal monitoring standards. *Anaesth Intens Care* **1988**; **16**: 110–3.
8 Eichhorn JH, Cooper JB, Cullen DJ, Maier WR, Philip JH, Seeman RG. Standards for patient monitoring during anesthesia at the Harvard Medical School *JAMA* 1986; **256**: 1017–20.
9 Block FE. We don't monitor enough. *J Clin Monit* 1986; **2**: 267–9.
10 Hamilton WK. Do we monitor enough? We monitor too much. *J Clin Monit* 1986; **2**: 264–6.
11 American Society of Anesthesiologists. Standards for basic intra-operative monitoring. In: *ASA Standards, Guidelines and Statements*. Philadelphia: ASA, October 1991.
12 Association of Anaesthetists of Great Britain and Ireland. *Recommendations for standards of monitoring during anaesthesia and recovery*. London: AAGBI, 1988 (revised 1995).
13 International Task Force on Anaesthesia Safety. International standards for a safe practice of anaesthesia. *Eur J Anaesth* 1993; **10** (Suppl. 7): 12–15.
14 Runciman WB, Webb RK, Lee R, Holland R. System failure: An analysis of 2000 incident reports. *Anaesth Intens Care* 1993; **21**: 684–95.
15 Webb RK, Van der Walt J, Runciman WB, Williamson JA, Cockings J, Russell WJ. Which monitor? A review of 2,000 anaesthetic incidents. *Anaesth Intens Care* 1993; **21**: 529–42.
16 Pearsall FJ, Davidson JA, Asbury AJ. Attitudes to the Association of Anaesthetists recommendations for standards of monitoring during anaesthesia and recovery. *Anaesthesia* 1995: **50**: 649–53.
17 Ludgate SM, Potter DC. European directives on medical devices. *BMJ* 1993; **307**: 459–60.

2 ECG monitoring

History

In the middle of the nineteenth century interest had been aroused in the so-called "action currents" detectable at the surface of the body when electrodes were placed upon the skin and means of detecting electrical currents applied to them. Action currents associated with cardiac activity were noted by Kolliker and Muller in 1856 and measurements made with an electrometer by Waller and Ludwig in 1887. The first serious measurements in human subjects were carried out by Einthoven[1] who used the string galvanometer, a device consisting of a quartz filament coated with metal suspended between the poles of an electromagnet and attached to the subject. The apparatus was crude by today's standards, but served to demonstrate that the tiny currents generated by cardiac activity could be translated into mechanical movement. The galvanometer was a popular instrument for the detection of small currents, since the torsion applied to the galvanometer "string" caused sufficient rotation to enable lightweight pointers to be moved on smoked paper wrapped on revolving drums in order to provide a permanent record. The use of ultraviolet light and ultraviolet-sensitive paper led to the attachment of mirrors to the galvanometer string. Reflection of light reaching the mirror by a short path along a longer pathway to the sensitive paper resulted in amplification of the movement owing the torsion of the string. Later, the advent of electronics enabled the electrical signals to be amplified directly. Now, the quality of the amplified signals was limited only by the difficulties of gaining and maintaining a satisfactory interface with the patient, in order to obtain unmodified signals from the subject, and the faithfulness with which the amplifiers of the day could reproduce the signal thus obtained.

Continuous ECG recording, or monitoring as we would call it now, seems to have appeared about 1920,[2] although its use in anaesthesia was heralded by Levy and Lewis in 1911,[3] when they noted the changes observable in the ECG during the course of chloroform anaesthesia. Although the regular use of the ECG for cardiac monitoring in the operating theatre was not to become commonplace until the early 1960s, a series of some 2500 cases was published in 1959.[4]

8

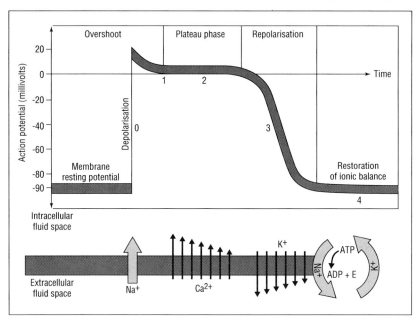

Figure 2.1 Cardiac action potential and ion flux. Diagrammatic representation of the electrical events in a cardiac cell. (0) depolarisation; (1) overshoot; (2) plateau; (3) repolarisation; (4) diastolic potential drift. Redrawn from Merrin RG. Cardiac cell membrane physiology: implications for the anesthesiologist. Current Opinion in Anesthesiology 1985;8:1–6; and Guidelines in Clinical Anaesthesiology 1985.

Theory

Depolarisation and repolarisation

The detectable electrical activity of the heart is based on the fact that both its conducting system and the cardiac muscle become depolarised on excitation and depolarised during recovery with each cardiac cycle (Figure 2.1).

Generation of action potentials in cardiac muscle

Action potentials have their origin in the transfer of ions across the cellular membranes of the heart, thereby changing the electrical potential on the respective surfaces of the membranes. During depolarisation, sodium ions rapidly enter myocardial cells followed by calcium. The normal "resting" potential is subsequently restored by an efflux of potassium ions from the cell. The excitation wave exhibits negative polarity as it flows

9

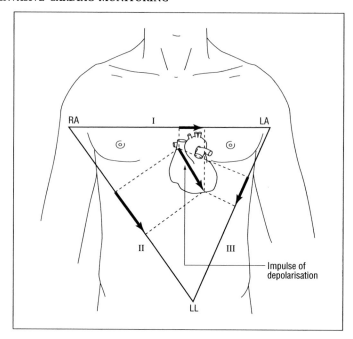

Figure 2.2 A sketch of Einthoven's triangle superimposed on the human torso, showing the relationship of the three bipolar leads (I, II and III) to the axis of electrical depolarisation in the heart.[B]

from the point of excitation, whereas repolarisation is characterised by positive polarity.

Transmission of the excitation wave by the conducting system

The depolarisation/repolarisation events give rise to potential differences which are transmitted to the surface of the body in the direction of their propagation within the heart (Figure 2.2). Hence, electrodes appropriately placed on the body surface can further conduct the electrical signals so generated and transmitted to them.

The cardiac impulse originates in the sinoatrial (S–A) node at the junction of the right atrium and right ventricle. From here it travels to the atrioventricular (A–V) node by way of internodal tracts of conducting tissue. From there it is conducted separately to the two ventricles via the bundle of His. The conducting system then divides into right and left bundle branches, the latter then dividing into anterior and posterior divisions (Figure 2.3).

10

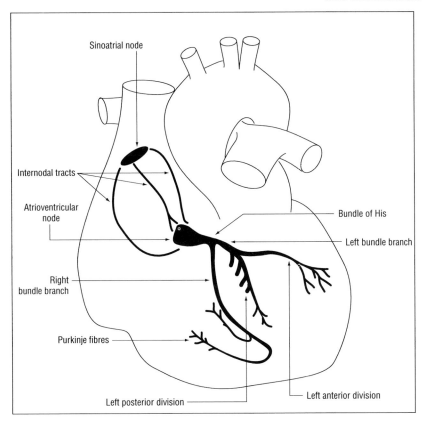

Figure 2.3 The conducting tissues of the heart.[A]

Further propagation through cardiac muscle

The various branches supply the adjacent muscle fibres and excite them. The excitation wave is therefore propagated through the myocardial muscle itself, producing potentials which, by reference to each other or to the sum of their effects, can be detected at the surface of the heart and, by further conduction through body tissues, at the surface of the body.

Coordinated contraction of cardiac muscle

Since the conducting system effectively coordinates myocardial contraction, the chambers of the normal heart may be expected to contract in a predictable manner described by the normal electrocardiogram (ECG). At any point in the myocardium, the propagated impulse, therefore, has direction and amplitude detectable via a surface electrode.

11

An electrode placed on the skin will receive conducted impulses with the polarity prevailing at the moment of reception. Should a pair of electrodes be placed some distance apart, any impulse approaching one of the pair as a wave of depolarisation will be negative with respect to the electrode from which it is flowing away. The signal acquired during the whole cycle will therefore describe the cardiac electrical events during that cardiac cycle and, when suitably amplified and displayed, constitute the ECG. It follows that the positioning of electrodes will reflect the amplitude, direction, and velocity of the electrical impulses concerned. The importance of positioning is exemplified by suggestions which have been made with a view to improving the quality of ECGs.[5] Moreover, the intended use of the electrode, e.g. in the coronary care unit, intensive care unit or operating theatre or for ambulatory monitoring, will influence the type selected.[6,7]

The electrodes are fixed at points which are both convenient and likely to reveal the pattern of greatest clinical interest. The time-honoured method, originally described by Einthoven and known as Einthoven's Triangle, is to affix them on the right arm (RA), left arm (LA) and left leg (LL). The connection between RA and LA is known as standard *Lead I*, that between RA and LL as *Lead II* and that between LA and LL as *Lead III* (Figure 2.4). In addition, the three leads are connected together in order to provide a point of reference for the potentials detected by the electrode pairs.

For diagnostic purposes, the 12-lead ECG is generally employed and, in addition to the three standard leads, consists of unipolar limb leads *aVR*, *aVL* and *aVF* and six unipolar chest (precordial) leads, V_1–V_6.

The term unipolar refers to the fact that only one electrode of a pair is used to detect an arriving impulse, the other serving only as a point of reference. The "a" in aVR, aVL and aVF denotes augmentation of the signal obtained from these electrodes, whilst the "R", "L" and "F" denote right (arm), left (arm) and (left) foot, respectively. The precordial leads are arranged across the anterior chest wall at predetermined sites, as shown.

Whenever detailed analysis of the ECG is required for diagnostic purposes, the 12-lead ECG should be invoked. However, for the purposes of this discussion, which concerns monitoring, certain lead combinations have been shown to confer advantages when early indications of myocardial disturbance are sought.

Amplification of the signal used to drive charts or displays

The signals of between 1 and 2 mV derived from electrodes and electrode pairs concerned in the derivation of the ECG are too small to power charting and display devices. Amplification is necessary. Figure 2.5 shows a diagrammatic representation of a typical electronic amplifier arrangement.

12

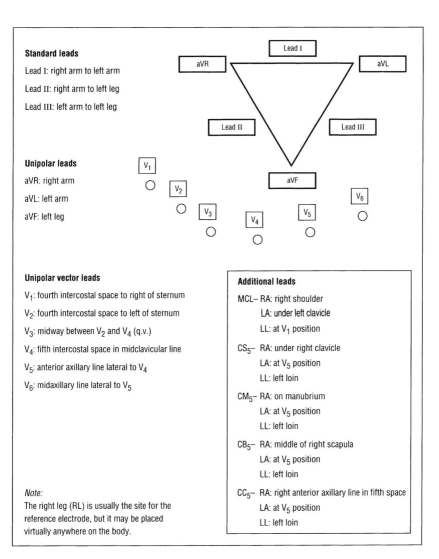

Figure 2.4 The 12-lead electrocardiogram and its important monitoring constituents.

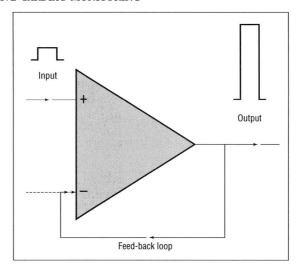

Figure 2.5 Diagrammatic representation of a simple amplifier. A signal, here a square wave, is supplied to the input and is amplified at the output. A fraction of the output signal is fed back to the input end of the amplifier at the point labelled negative (−), showing that it is then inverted with respect to the form of the signal at the normal signal input (+), to offset internal distortion during amplification and promote linearity. In the event that electrostatic or electromagnetic interference should affect the input, the amplifier may be so arranged that these interfering signals affect both negative (inverting) and positive (non-inverting) inputs, shown as broken and unbroken lines, respectively, and cancel each other out, effectively leaving only the monitored signal applied at the non-inverted input (+) to be amplified for output.

Certain factors are important in the amplification of signals and these are well demonstrated by the problems posed by ECG signals. In order to amplify the ECG signals faithfully, i.e. without distortion, the amplifier should have good performance in respect of at least the following characteristics:

- linearity
- absence of drift
- noise (interference) rejection.

Amplitude linearity

It is essential that the amplifier be capable of amplifying all received signals to the same degree. That is to say, if the values of the input signals are plotted against the values of the corresponding output signals, the resultant plot should be as close as possible to a straight line.

14

Gain stability

The ECG signal may be amplified to different levels, i.e. $\times 2$, $\times 3$, etc. The extent of amplification should be consistent at each level. However, it is unusual to require large ranges of amplification for this signal, in contrast with the range of amplification levels required, for example, in blood pressure measurement, where there may be a requirement to display the trace or record it at a variety of levels.

Drift

A much less serious problem nowadays, drift is the phenomenon by which the value of the output departs from the original calibration value with the passage of time. The design and components of modern amplifiers render this an almost negligible factor.

Suitable frequency response

The frequency band occupied by the ECG is 0–100 Hz. The amplifier must be capable of maintaining linearity and freedom from drift over this range and, in practice, this is easily attained. It should be noted, however, that the mains supply frequency of 50 Hz is at the middle of this range, so that it may be expected that the mains supply will be a major factor in electrical interference.

Noise rejection

Noise is the term used to describe unwanted signals which find their way into the signal detection and amplification system. It may arise from a number of sources.

Electrostatic interference

The basis of electrostatic interference is that under certain circumstances, a subject may come within the sphere of influence of a fluctuating electrical field such as that due to the alternating (AC) mains current flowing along a nearby mains cable. The 50 Hz mains frequency sets up a surrounding fluctuating field which induces an opposite charge on the patient. It consequently injects a spurious signal which interferes with the normally generated biological potentials. The interference from such sources may be substantial and such as to overwhelm the signals of interest as they are

15

passed to the amplifier. In addition to these more obvious sources, the patient may pick up interference by virtue of forming one element of what is in effect a capacitor: for example, patient and operating table, or patient and bed or couch. These stray capacitances are added to the signals of interest and distort them.

Electromagnetic interference

Mains current, as has been stated, generates a changing electromagnetic field around any conductor along which it passes. The effect is known as inductance.

In turn, this changing field will induce a corresponding current in any conductor, such as a lead carrying an ECG signal, with the 50 Hz frequency of the mains supply. This is superimposed on the signal of interest and constitutes mains interference. Similarly, any such changing electromagnetic field may affect conducting pathways within the amplifier itself.

Electromagnetic disturbance may be also be caused by other apparatus which generate fluctuating electrical fields, such as electric motors, electrical and electronic switches, diathermy,[8] radio frequency equipment (especially that equipped with antennae, such as radiocommunication and radiotelephony equipment), and computing equipment. It is essential that, in critical applications, the *emitting* device or the *susceptible* device be suitably shielded, whilst many medical amplifiers are now designed specifically to minimise interference due to diathermy.

The more general implications of a recently published European Union Directive on electromagnetic compatibility have been reviewed concisely,[9] whilst the medical requirements are contained in IEC Standards and their European equivalents.[10–12]

The effects of electrostatic and electromagnetic interference (Figure 2.6) may be minimised by shielding the apparatus and any conducting leads in a metal sheath (flexible for the leads), attached to the casing of the instrument or to a common reference point, so that the effect of all such currents is cancelled out. In the case of electromagnetic interference, connecting leads need to be shielded in a twisted pair of cables such that the potential in the shielding wire is the obverse of that in the lead (achieved by inverting the interfering signal). Such action may not be sufficient, in which case the input of the amplifier may need to be arranged so that the aggregation of signals other than the signal of interest is fed into the input in an inverted form. Thus the two signals, the interference signal and the inverted interference signal, cancel each other.

The signal representing this aggregated interference is drawn from an electrode or electrodes placed well away from the path of the signal under scrutiny. In the case of the ECG, an *indifferent* lead on RL would be placed

16

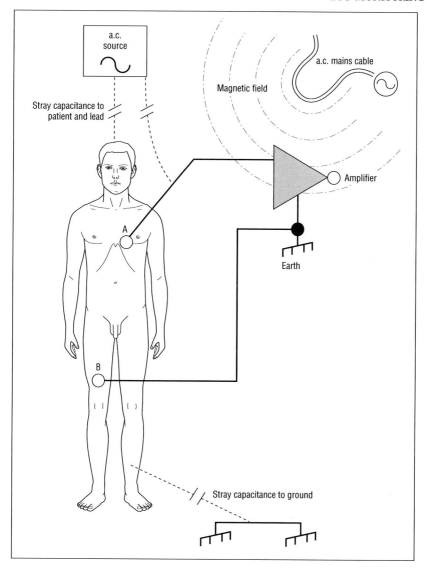

Figure 2.6 A simple amplifier subject to interference from electrostatic (broken lines) and electromagnetic sources.[C]

sufficiently far away from the RA and LL of Lead II, for example. The extent to which the amplifier is capable of eliminating the effects of the interfering signal in this way is referred to as the common mode rejection ratio. It should be better than 1000:1 and is usually considerably better.

17

Matching

When more than one amplifier is present in a monitoring array, it is necessary for the output of each to be compatible with the input of others to which it is connected. Modules from the same manufacturer, especially when supplied as modules in a standard common housing, are likely to be compatible, but care should be exercised when free-standing items from different sources are coupled together. However, some amplifiers are able to sense the level and quality of their inputs and adjust them accordingly.

Electrode potentials

Electrodes, unless made of specially chosen materials, may interact with moisture and salt at the point of contact with the body to produce polarisation and, hence, distortion of the signals sensed at that point. Electrodes constructed so as to avoid this effect are said to be *reversible electrodes*.

Electrode impedance

The effects of impedance make a significant contribution to interference. It has already been stated that interference due to current induced in leads may be limited by adequate shielding. However, if the shielding is inadequate, the amplitude of the interfering signal may be greater than the signal being detected at the skin surface and conducted by the lead to the amplifier. The electrode itself may exacerbate this by acting as a high impedance if, for example, local contact is poor and it effectively forms a capacitor with the skin. A significant protection is offered by ensuring that the amplifier has a *high input impedance*.

Earth loops

When more than one item of electrical equipment is connected to the patient, as when there is another item of monitoring or therapeutic equipment attached, these may carry charges at differing potentials. Commonly, this is attributable to connection to earth at widely spaced points, such that the earth potential is not constant throughout the supply

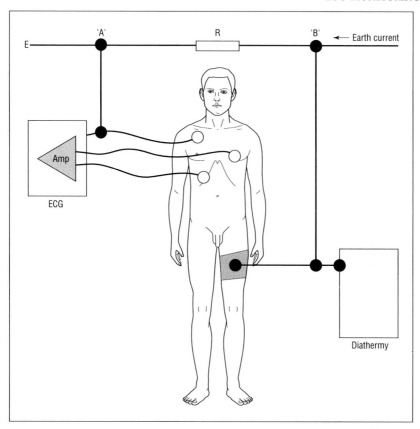

Figure 2.7 Interference due to an earth loop between points A and B. An earth current (usually due to earth leakage from some other device attached to the earth) sets up a potential difference across the small resistance R. This potential gradient across the patient is detected by the amplifier (AMP) and appears as interference.[C]

system (Figure 2.7). This potential difference will be consistently present and added to the signals of interest. The solution is, where possible and when earthing is required, to choose a common earthing point, such as a single mains supply socket.

Calibration and maintenance

Although amplifiers in much current medical equipment, including ECGs, are of high quality, it is essential that manufacturers' instructions concerning calibration and routine maintenance of the equipment containing them are followed. This is of particular importance where ECG

19

equipment is used outside institutions with routine maintenance facilities, for example in general practice surgeries.

Preferred lead arrangements

CM$_5$ (and CB$_5$) in cardiac monitoring

Lead II and leads CM$_5$ and CB$_5$ are of particular value in cardiac monitoring. Lead II roughly corresponds with the normal cardiac axis and may, as part of a simple 3-lead ECG, reveal arrhythmias or give an indication of myocardial ischaemia.[13] It has long been favoured by anaesthetists for this reason. The CM$_5$ lead is bipolar and connects the manubrium and the V$_5$ positions. It is said to permit ready identification and discrimination of arrhythmias and to assist in the recognition of most instances of left ventricular ischaemia.[14] The electrodes are easy to apply in these positions and the positions are readily maintained. It is accessible during anaesthesia and is favoured during general anaesthesia when arrhythmias and ischaemia are among the greatest threats to the patient's well-being.

The CB$_5$ lead, which is again a bipolar lead, in this case connecting the right scapular area with the V$_5$ position, enhances the P and Q waves, again making the detection of arrhythmias and ischaemia easier.[15,16] Despite the advantages claimed for this lead arrangement, which is eminently suitable for erect and sitting patients, the relative inaccessibility and susceptibility to disturbance of the scapular position limit its use in anaesthesia and critical care.

Vector leads (V$_{1-6}$)

The unipolar precordial[17] vector leads have a special place when specific parts of the heart are under scrutiny. In monitoring applications this is less likely than is the case in a diagnostic clinic. Nevertheless V$_5$, in particular, is regarded as a good lead for the identification of left ventricular ischaemia and, indeed, is preferred by some to the CM$_5$ lead[18,19] and to the rather more invasive oesophageal lead[20,21] (Figure 2.8).

Electrodes

The purpose of electrodes is to permit the transfer of the very small electrical signals presenting at the surface of the skin to the ECG sensing and recording system. Good conductivity is essential, whilst any gaps or foreign materials which are poor conductors of electricity will degrade the

20

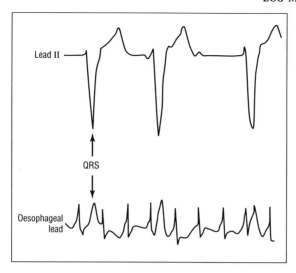

Figure 2.8 Comparison of a trace from lead II (above) with an oesophageal trace (below) in a patient with atrial fibrillation[B], and Kates RA, Zaidan JR, Kaplan JA. Esophageal lead for intraoperative electrocardiographic monitoring. Anesth Analg 1982; 61: 781–5.

quality of the signal. The larger the surface area of the electrodes, the better the chances of avoiding degradation. However, a balance must be struck between the ideal and other considerations such as surface occupancy, methods of attachment, and cost.

Materials

Metal plates have long been favoured for high quality ECG recording. When used as limb lead plates, they have the advantage of a large area of contact with the skin. The usual method of attachment is by encircling, often elastic, bands which are very effective in keeping the plates in position. Traditionally, they have been used with leads with the use of quite large pins inserted into equally large terminals on the plates. They are thus inconvenient for continuous use in patients who are conscious or fully awake. They have been largely supplanted by miniature electrodes consisting of a small metal pad, usually overlaid by a thin foam layer impregnated with a suitable conductive gel. The materials most commonly used are silver and silver chloride, the metal and salt coating being such as to minimise electrolytic activity and subsequent polarisation of the electrode. The plates themselves are very small and thin and the gel relatively abundant, so that distortion of the skin produces little disturbance to the signal. The whole is mounted on an adhesive patch through which a thin electric lead passes to a miniature lead socket or upon which is mounted

21

Electrodes – apparatus and precautions

Choice of electrodes

- Select plates or electrodes with due consideration for their use in monitoring.
- Look for the greatest area of patient contact consistent with ease of use.
- Are they easy to attach and easy to secure?
- If adhesive, do they adhere for a reasonable length of time?
- Are they easily dislodged in the monitoring setting under review?

Nature of the interface

- Think of what can interfere with signal transmission.
- Is the skin well hydrated? If not, its impedance may be changed and it may conduct less well.

Electrode attachment

- Take care when applying the electrodes – good contact improves performance.
- Attach the electrodes securely. If they are self-adhesive, prepare the skin as instructed.

Cleansing and preparation of skin

- The contact you will achieve is only as good as the skin surface presented. In many monitoring settings, e.g. in intensive care, the skin will have received special attention continually. Elsewhere, the skin may be soiled, crusty, greasy, etc. If so, prepare it accordingly. Abrasion of the skin is unnecessary.
- Ensure that any medium (cream, jelly, or gel) is appropriate to your monitoring application.

Care of leads

- ECG monitoring leads are often rather fragile. Do not place them under undue stress from stretching, kinking, etc. Keep leads short to minimise interference.
- Make sure that any lead cable run is clear of sharp edges and does not allow the cable to become entrapped in cot sides, drawers and the like.

Connecting up – significance of colour coding

- Make sure your leads are connected properly and securely. If the leads are colour coded, make sure the colour coding system is the same as that used by the ECG monitor. They are not necessarily the same. If in doubt look for the markings (e.g. RA, LA, LL).

a press stud lead terminal. Although some of the early examples were supplied with poor adhesive and were prone to easy dislodgement, many current examples are quite satisfactory, the types with the press stud terminal being especially popular.

Conductive medium

An amazing range of proprietary creams, jellies, and gels has been available to provide the interface between electrode and skin when this is necessary to maintain a satisfactory contact and good conduction. It has been shown on many occasions that other substances, ranging from tomato ketchup and salad cream to saline solution will do the job.[22] Nevertheless, convenience, aesthetic considerations, and reliability render the dedicated compounds a prudent choice. The advent of disposable electrodes with pads impregnated with a suitable gel has largely eliminated the need for separate conductive media.

Electrode impedance

The size and characteristics of electrodes is of importance in relation to the impedance encountered at the point of contact between electrode and skin. It will be remembered that Ohm's law relates electromotive force (emf) to current and resistance as $E = IR$, where the emf is expressed in volts, current in amperes, and resistance in ohms. However, this holds true only for direct current. When the current is alternating, then the effects of capacitance (C) and inductance (L) must be taken into account. Both capacitance and inductance are a function of the frequency of the current, and the manifestations of opposition to current flow occasioned by them are known as their capacitative reactance (X_C) and inductive reactance (X_L), respectively. Their combined effects, together with that of pure resistance R, is the impedance (Z) expressed in ohms. The resultant impedance is significant and is generally dealt with by providing the ECG amplifier with high input impedance.

Electrode–skin potentials

Small potentials are created by the epidermis and by the battery-like electrochemical cell effect of the electrode–skin combination. These amount to some 25 mV and fall within a narrow range, so that a band-pass filter covering 20–30 mV should eradicate the problem.

23

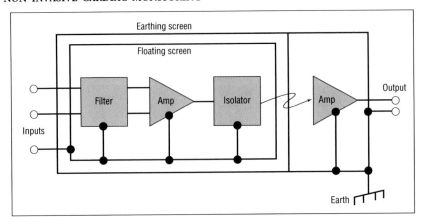

Figure 2.9 The principles of a diathermy-immune ECG amplifier (AMP=amplifier).[c]

Patient isolation

It is important, for reasons of safety and for the further reduction of interference, to prevent currents induced in or applied to patients (for example, from diathermy earth-proving currents) from passing to earth by way of the ECG leads. Should the unwanted currents pass through the heart, they may result in "microshock", a phenomenon in which small currents of 10–100 μA may incite serious arrhythmias such as ventricular fibrillation. To this end, equipment should be isolated from the mains supply by a transformer or some other means of achieving physical electrical discontinuity.

Similarly, the input to the ECG amplifier and lead system may be isolated from the mains current by a transformer, whose windings pass the required signals by mutual induction, but prevent certain other currents from passing or, better, by optoelectronic isolation (Figure 2.9). In this mode, a photoemitting device, usually a photodiode, transmits the ECG signal to a photoelectric receiving cell, thereby avoiding electrical continuity altogether. More advanced methods have appeared, including adaptive noise filtering, in which digitisation of the incoming signals enables the ECG signal to be differentiated from interference.

Specifications for the design of ECGs in general, and for monitoring ECGs in particular, are given in standards prepared by the International Electrotechnical Commission (IEC).[23,24] Where such monitors are combined with defibrillation equipment, special considerations apply.[25]

24

Display and recording conventions

When a paper record of the ECG is made, the horizontal time axis is calibrated on a scale of $0.04\,\text{s mm}^{-1}$ and the vertical axis is calibrated in steps of $0.1\,\text{mV mm}^{-1}$. A choice of paper speeds may be available.

When the ECG is displayed as a trace on a screen, for example a cathode-ray tube (CRT) or a liquid crystal display (LCD) panel, the horizontal (time) axis is handled as continuous left-to-right sweep and the vertical axis calibrated at $10\,\text{mV cm}^{-1}$. A choice of trace sweep speeds may be available.

Deflections correspond to changes in the amplitude and direction of the cardiac impulse, as sensed by a single electrode or as the potential difference between two electrodes.

Cardiac axis

Determination

Limb leads

The cardiac axis may be determined in a rough and ready manner by consideration of the limb leads. In each of the limb lead traces, there are positive- and negative-going portions of the QRS trace for each cardiac cycle. The lead with the most prominent positive (or up-going) QRS component indicates the lead aligned approximately with the axis of the heart. When the assessment has to be made from a monitoring trace on a transient display such as a CRT, or is determined from a strip taken from monitoring leads, this method is quick and consistent with the imperfections of the monitoring setting.

Vector leads

A better estimate of the cardiac axis may be obtained from a consideration of the vector leads. Here, vectors are drawn on a diagram, such that they can be resolved into a single resultant vector indicative of the cardiac axis (Figure 2.10). Whilst the method may be used in conjunction with a hard copy recording of ECG monitoring output, it is less easily derived from a displayed trace. The significance of the determination of the cardiac axis lies in its correlation with enlargement, either dilatation or hypertrophy, of the chambers of the heart, especially of the right and left ventricles. However, it is the resultant of a number of factors, including hypertrophy in one or more chambers, contributing to what is, after all, simply a summation of the corresponding electrical signals detected by a lead or

25

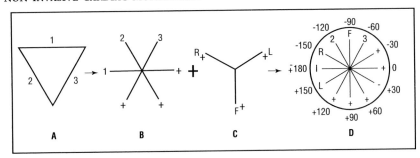

Figure 2.10 (A) Einthoven's triangle, the sides of which represent the three standard limb leads; (B) The reference system composed of the three sides of Einthoven's triangle rearranged so that they bisect one another; (C) Lines of derivation of the three unipolar (aV) limb leads; (D) The reference system composed of lines of derivation of the six limb leads (B + C) arranged so they bisect each other[B] and Marriott HJL. Practical electrocardiography, ed. 6. Baltimore: Williams & Wilkins 1977.

lead pair. It must, therefore, be interpreted in the light of other ECG and related findings during monitoring.

ECG waveform

Derivation

The propagated electrical waves due to the excitation of the cardiac conducting system and the contracting myocardial cells produce signals at the surface of the body which, as has been stated, may be detected by means of suitably placed electrodes and electrode pairs. When these signals are amplified and fed to a display or recorder, they result in a pattern of changes of amplitude (on the y-axis) which take place with respect to time (on the x-axis). In the case of displays such as CRTs and LCD panels, this is achieved by having the trace sweep from left to right. Thus, they provide a time base on the x-axis commensurate with the rate of cardiac activity and which at the same time yields a pattern recognisable as the ECG.

Chart recorders achieve the same objective by moving the paper recording strip at a speed commensurate with the calibrations implied by the grid pattern imprinted on it.

Elements

The normal ECG (Figure 2.11) consists of a number of distinguishable elements resulting from its variation in amplitude against the defined timebase. The commonly described elements are the P-wave, the QRS complex and the T-wave.

26

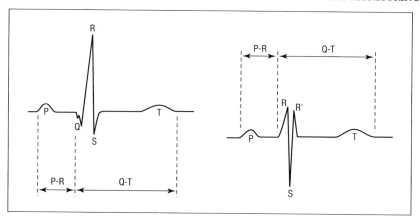

Figure 2.11 The normal ECG pattern with its component parts (as described in the text)[A] and Guidelines in Clinical Anaesthesia 1985.

P-wave

The P-wave is the electrical expression of the contraction of the right atrium. Since it is travelling from the S–A node to the A–V node it provides a positive deflection in Lead I. The normal amplitude is of the order of 2·5 mm, and a P-wave taller than this may indicate right atrial hypertrophy.

P–R interval

The P–R interval describes the interval between the beginning of the P-wave and the beginning of the R-wave. The duration of the P–R interval should be no less than 0·12 s and no greater than 0·2 s. Intervals greater than this indicate some kind of conduction defect.

QRS complex

The QRS complex consists of a brief and usually small negative deflection (Q), immediately followed by a positive deflection (R), which is then followed by a positive deflection (T) of variable amplitude and duration. The extent of the deflection representing the Q-wave is variable, but deep Q-waves are generally of serious import, often reflecting ischaemic change such as an old or recent myocardial infarction.

The R-wave represents right ventricular contraction and its amplitude is dependent upon the position of the electrode or electrode pair from which the particular signal is derived. This is best seen in the unipolar vector leads, where there is normally a progressive increase in the amplitude of the deflection from V_1 to V_4, followed by a decline in V_5 and V_6.

The S-wave represents left ventricular contraction and is best seen in the unipolar vector leads towards the left of the precordium, i.e. V_4 to V_6. Its normal maximum height in the vector leads is some 25 mm.

The combined height of the tallest R-wave and the tallest S-wave, if exceeding 35 mm, suggests left ventricular hypertrophy, which may be corroborated by a negative deflection in lead aVL greater than 11 mm. The duration of the QRS complex should not exceed 0·12 s.

S–T interval

The S–T interval, timed from the end of the S-wave to the onset of the T-wave, represents the interval between the completion of contraction and the beginning of depolarisation.

T-wave

The T-wave represents depolarisation of the myocardium. Its duration is variable and its height is influenced by a number of factors. Generally speaking, conditions which reduce the excitability of cardiac muscle, such as hypocalcaemia and hyperkalaemia, reduce its amplitude, whilst hypercalcaemia increases it.

Other significant elements

The only other feature worthy of mention here is the U-wave. It follows the T-wave and may continue directly from it. It is concerned with repolarisation and may or may not be evident, and often accompanies clinical hypothermia. It is an inconstant feature.

ECG strip chart output

Required characteristics

ECG strip recorders may be modules in monitoring arrays. However, the majority are stand-alone instruments used in differing circumstances. If the device is portable, it should be sufficiently rugged to withstand the treatment it is likely to receive.

28

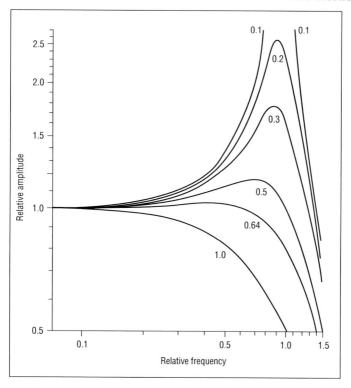

Figure 2.12 Amplitude distortion with increasing frequency. The number by each curve is the damping factor (D). D= 1·0 represents critical damping, D= 0.1 is undamped. When D= 0·64 the recorded amplitude is accurate to within ± 2% up to about two thirds of the undamped natural frequency.[C]
(Relative frequency = fraction of undamped frequency).

Distortions

Pen recorders and ultraviolet recorders using mirrors may be subject to certain distortions of the ECG waveform. The most important are amplitude, phase, sine and tangential distortions.

Amplitude distortion

Amplitude distortion (Figure 2.12) is evident when a writing arm is required to operate at increasing frequencies of oscillation. Because it has mass, it acquires momentum and has a tendency to overshoot. The system has a resonant frequency, referable to the mass of the arm and the tension of the spring which is designed to return it to the base line, such as to produce the greatest overshoot at that frequency. The performance of the arm can be improved by making it as light as possible and by using a spring with relatively high tension, so that the mass of the arm is small by

29

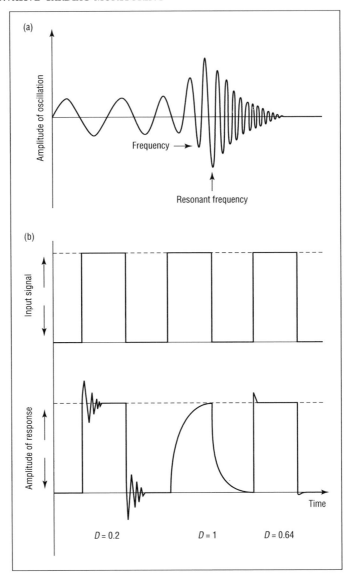

Figure 2.13 (a) Effect of increasing frequency on amplitude of recorded signal with constant amplitude sine wave input; (b) Response to square wave input. Left: minimal damping showing overshoot and oscillation. Centre: critically damped (overshoot just abolished). Right: damping 64% of critical showing maximum speed of response with minimal overshoot. D = damping factor.[C]

comparison. Alternatively, damping may be applied, by applying an electrically generated or mechanical opposing force. The damping may provided by, for example, viscous fluid loading of the galvanometer or inductive opposition to movement. Damping (Figure 2.13) is critical when all overshoot is removed. This, however, may provide excessive hindrance to the movement required to reproduce the signal faithfully. A more satisfactory degree of damping is afforded at some 65% of this level, when it is said to be optimal and permits the best frequency response in practice. Damping is expressed in terms of the damping factor (D), where $D=1$ for critical damping. Over- and underdamping are reflected in values > and <1, respectively. Optimal damping therefore corresponds to a damping factor of 0·65.

If the frequency is increased still further the arm is unable to keep up with the frequency of oscillation required of it and describes a decreasing oscillation about the baseline as the signal frequency rises. Fortunately, this last activity occurs at frequencies above those encountered in ECG monitoring and is only of importance when small transients are being followed for detailed diagnostic purposes.

Phase distortion

Phase distortion (Figure 2.14) is similarly caused by the mass of the writing arm and the inertia which has to be overcome each time it is accelerated from the point of reversal. The result is a delay such that the peak of the trace is written to the paper shortly after the true point on the paper has moved on. The writing point is displaced from the perpendicular to the time-base by an angle which, at the resonant frequency of the system, is 90°. Again, damping may improve the situation, optimal damping being most appropriate.

Sine distortion

Sine distortion (Figure 2.15) is the aberration in the written trace which occurs as a result of the pen arm having to describe an arc about its fulcrum, rather than travelling perpendicularly to the trace base line. The error becomes more significant with larger excursions of the arm, since the early part of its travel is close to the perpendicular whereas, with (excessively) large swings, it is increasingly veering away from it. The arc described by the pen arm has a length of $r\theta$ radians, where r is the length of the arm and, hence, the radius r of the arc and θ is the angle the arm makes with the base line neutral position at maximum deflection (Figure 2.16).

As can be seen in the figure, the distance from the base line when the pen comes to rest at the maximum deflection is less than would have been the case had the trace been perpendicular to the base line. The sine error

31

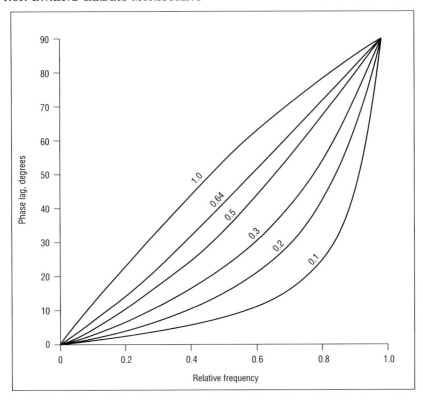

Figure 2.14 Phase lag with increasing frequency, D=1 represents critical damping, D=0·1 is underdamped. Phase lag is proportional to frequency when D=0·64. (Relative frequency=fraction of undamped natural frequency).[C]

has the value r sine θ. It is also displaced backwards. The delay this causes in writing on the moving paper is the timing error t of $r - r \cos \theta$.

Tangential distortion

Tangential distortion (Figure 2.17) is peculiar to recorders in which the heat-sensitive paper passes over a knife-edge over which a lengthened heated stylus sweeps with each complex (Figure 2.18). This method was introduced in the first place as a means of overcoming the timing error already referred to, but introduces an error of its own. Here, the fact that at maximum excursion the point of contact is further along the elongated stylus and, hence, along the arm, exaggerates the amplitude of the trace. The greater the excursion the greater is the degree of exaggeration. The error in this instance is $r \tan \theta$.

32

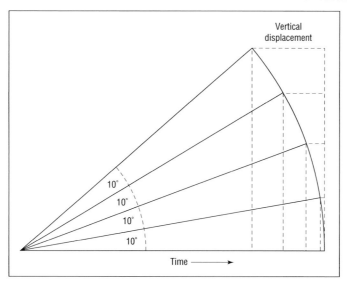

Figure 2.15 Angular displacements of writing arm of 10°, 20°, 30°, and 40° to show relative magnitudes of sine error and timing with 10 cm long arm.[C]

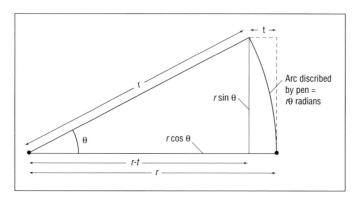

Figure 2.16 Sources of distortion in a pen recorder. The pen (of length r) describes an arc whose length is rθ radians. The vertical displacement of the pen tip is r sin θ and timing error is t = r − r cos θ. The sine error causes the vertical displacement to be less than it should be at large angular displacements.[C]

CRT displays and LCD panels

CRT displays

The cathode ray oscilloscope tube (CRT) employs a high velocity electron beam which interacts with a high-persistence phosphor coating to produce a glowing spot on the screen (Figure 2.19).

33

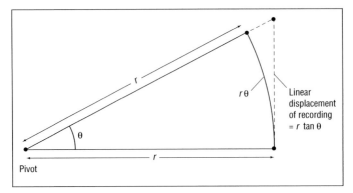

Figure 2.17 Tangent error which must be corrected in recorders using knife edge and heated stylus, ink-jet or mirror galvanometers. The error in the vertical displacement gets larger as the angular displacement increases.[C]

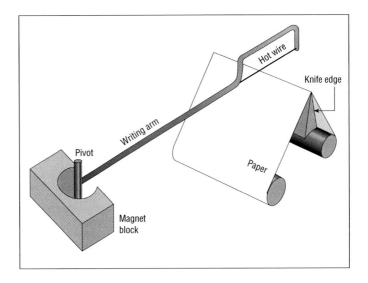

Figure 2.18 Use of knife-edge and heated stylus to overcome timing error.[C]

The beam is deflected in two planes at right angles to each other, horizontal and vertical, the deflection being caused by the placing of paired plates in each plane across which there is an electrical potential. The horizontal deflection corresponds to the x-axis of a plot and the vertical to the y-axis. The potential applied to the horizontal plate is a constantly rising voltage (or ramp voltage) such as to draw the beam from a biased position at the left of the screen, followed by a return of the bias voltage such as to cause the return of the beam to its starting position at the left of the screen. The x-axis thus forms a time-base for the ECG trace and is

34

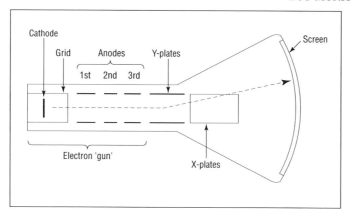

Figure 2.19 Cathode Ray Tube (CRT).[c]

calibrated accordingly. The vertical deflection is centred upon the *x*-axis which is itself placed in a position on the screen convenient for viewing. The potential on this *y*-axis is the amplified signal obtained from the ECG leads. Hence, the *y*-axis trace oscillates in concert with the ECG potential, whilst the movement on the *x*-axis elongates this oscillation into the familiar ECG pattern. The analogue signal is therefore displayed by analogue means. High definition is possible but, for monitoring purposes, visibility may take precedence over discrimination.

An indication of heart rate may be derived from the ECG signal. Errors may arise when other parts of the ECG waveform are of an amplitude close to that of the R-wave and are spuriously detected and counted, as may be bifid R-waves. The monitor may be designed to avoid such errors, but may not succeed in eliminating them. Arrhythmias present similar difficulties, as does a drifting electrical baseline. The analogue ECG signal may be digitised, i.e. the analogue signal is sampled at very close intervals and the discrete value at each point held as amplitude data. The benefits of this approach include the ability to relay the signal in digital format to other instruments for display recording and analysis or to processing the signal there and then within the ECG apparatus. This is of significance in ECG monitoring, in that trends may be assessed and arrhythmias and other important disorders identified by software algorithms. Thus, automatic processing and interpretation has become practicable and is limited largely by the skill and experience reflected in the quality of the pertinent algorithms.

Other features important in ECG monitoring include the ability to "freeze" digitally based displays so that they, in effect, stand still for closer examination and processing so that instead of the ECG pattern travelling across the display screen in conjunction with the time-base, the time-base itself travels backwards, yielding the impression of a continuously backward moving ECG trace; latest new ECG complexes appear successively at the

35

right-hand edge of the display. Samples of the trace obtained over a limited period may be stored for examination and analysis later. Further, multiple displays of the same ECG trace may be presented, one of which may be "frozen" or presented in a different format for accentuation of given features. Where the ECG is displayed with other variables and their parameters, such as blood pressures or respiratory traces, colour is often used for better discrimination of the traces of each of the displayed variables.

LCD panels

LCD panels also use a digitised version of the ECG signal, each digital value of which is conducted to a specific point (*pixel*) in a two-dimensional display matrix. The definition achievable is a function of the arrangement of the display matrix. Hitherto, the speed with which individual pixels could be illuminated and extinguished placed a limit on the definition of the trace as seen by the viewer, some "ghosting" often being apparent. Current displays are, however, sufficiently responsive for this not to be a serious problem. Again, many of the advanced features of digital CRTs are available, including freezing, storage, processing and, in the latest models, colour. A major advantage possessed by LCD, gas-discharge, and similar panel displays is the much reduced current drain on battery power supplies. They are thus likely to be found in portable ECG display equipment.

Effects of interference

Some forms of interference are immediately apparent on a CRT display. For example, the 50 Hz interference from the mains, provided it does not swamp the trace, appears as a fine superimposed oscillation. Despite its presence, a trace that would be unacceptable for cardiological investigation may be sufficiently clear for monitoring purposes.

Choosing a suitable instrument

The longest and most impressive specification may be more demanding than the monitoring application merits and *vice versa*. The important points to be borne in mind concern the suitability of the ECG monitor or recorder for the envisaged monitoring application(s). In particular, it should be suitable for the electrical environment in which it is to be used. The characteristics required of amplifiers for ECG monitoring have been described (q.v.) and the American Heart Association[26] has published specifications which include a linear frequency response between 0·14 and

Minimising interference with ECG monitoring displays and recorders and maintaining their performance

Environment

- Avoid "hostile" electrical environments, where there is diathermy, diagnostic or therapeutic X-ray equipment, electrical generators, where possible.
- Make sure you use a common earthing point for earthed equipment (where possible, use a single mains socket outlet). Remember the possibility of earth loops when more than one monitoring or therapeutic device is connected to the subject.
- Keep monitoring leads as short as may be practicable and keep them away from mains cables and other sources of electrostatic charge and mutual induction.

Choice of equipment

Recent types of recorder use a stylus or ink jet in a head moving truly perpendicularly to the path of the paper. Both sine and tangential distortion are thus eliminated. Ink-jet heads are capable of handling frequencies well in excess of those demanded for faithful ECG reproduction, whereas the arm-mounted stylus may be close to its working limits.

Minimisation of distortion

The elongated heated stylus writing on heat-sensitive paper was introduced to obviate timing errors. Other methods involved special linkages to enable the stylus to follow a path perpendicular to the paper and placement of the writing arm perpendicular to the paper which ran in a trough whose shape corresponded with the arc traversed by the arm. The important point for prospective users is to know whether these errors are present and whether any attempts have been made to reduce or overcome them.

- Make sure that your ECG equipment is suitably protected against electrical interference, i.e. that its susceptibility is minimised by shielding, appropriate design of amplifiers, etc.
- By the same token, check whether or not your ECG, or any modules with which it is housed in common, may emit radiation which could interfere with other important equipment. Is it protected in any way to minimize these effects?
- Buy good quality leads, especially when choosing replacements or disposable types.
- Buy good quality electrodes – the cheapest are not necessarily the best, although some of the best are also among the most competitive.
- When choosing ECG monitoring displays and recorders, make sure that the equipment is suitable for the application(s) you have in mind and the environment in which it will need to be operated (e.g. hospital or home; CCU, ICU or clinic; general practice surgery; community site; or the home). Will it be transported and be subjected to the shocks and vibration of being carried in a vehicle?

50 Hz. However, given that monitoring often takes place in hospital electrical environments, in which it may be impractical to avoid having mains cables and other potent sources of interference in the vicinity, a bandwidth falling short of the 50 Hz mains frequency, say 0·5–40 Hz, permits reasonable appreciation of important abnormalities, whilst eliminating some of the more troublesome forms of interference. The sources of hazards, including interference, their nature and reasonable precautions to be taken, have been reviewed by Hull.[27]

Training

The ECG is now sufficiently commonplace in institutions for it to be taken for granted that all concerned are familiar with it. As a result, and all too frequently, ECG monitors are set up with insufficient thought for those who must respond to them. It is not satisfactory that an ECG monitor be placed at the bedside of a patient in a general hospital ward and a junior night nurse requested to "keep an eye on it" without any instruction in the function of the instrument, the information it is expected to convey, or the response which is expected. A recent report from the Medical Devices Agency[28] sets out clearly the circumstances under which monitoring devices should be used. It is essential that those who set up and have care of such equipment are properly trained in its use and are fully briefed for a particular application.[29]

Complications of ECG monitoring

Like all monitoring techniques, ECG monitoring can be associated with hazard or mishap. Indeed, some hazards arise from the very prevalence of the technique and the fact that familiarity readily breeds contempt.

Commoner complications

- ECG monitors which are mains operated are subject to the usual *hazards of medical electrical equipment*, especially if not properly and regularly maintained, and if the operators are not trained in the use of the equipment. Manuals are, of course, provided with these instruments, but are rarely available or read.
- *Electrocution* may result from
  - faulty earthing of earthed apparatus;
  - faulty insulation;

- damaged mains cables (caught in cot-sides and bedside table drawers);
- damage from repeated dragging on the cable when the plug itself should be removed from its socket;
- being run over by sundry vehicles and trolleys.
- *Burns* may be sustained in circumstances where diathermy currents are able to find a path to earth by way of ECG monitoring leads. These can be prevented by careful attention to the application of diathermy apparatus to the patient according to its type and by using patient-isolated monitoring equipment.
- *Personal injury* to patient or operator may be caused by poorly supported equipment, given that ECG monitoring may be required virtually anywhere.
- Inexperience in the use of the instrument may result in *unsatisfactory traces or recordings* when the availability of vital information would have enabled prompt and correct action to be taken.

Prevention

Means of prevention may be very briefly summarised[30]:

- appropriate choice of equipment;
- proper maintenance;
- training of users.

1 Einthoven W. Le telecardiogramme. *Arch Int Physiol* 1906; **4**: 132–64.
2 Lennox WG, Graves RC, Levine SA. An electrocardiographic study of fifty patients during operation. *Arch Intern Med* 1922; **30**: 57–72.
3 Levy AG, Lewis T. Heart irregularities resulting from the inhalation of low percentages of chloroform vapour, and their relationship to ventricular fibrillation. *Heart* 1911; **3**: 99–112.
4 Katz AM. Mechanisms of disease: cardiac ion channels. *N Engl J Med* 1993; **328**: 1244–51.
5 Herman MV, Ingram DA, Levy JA, Cook JR, Athans RJ. Variability of electrocardiographic precordial lead placement: a method to improve accuracy and reliability. *Clin Cardiol* 1991; **14**: 469–76.
6 ANSI/AAMI. *American National Standard for pregelled ECG disposable electrodes*. American Standards Institute (ANSI) and Association for the Advancement of Medical Instrumentation (AAMI), 1984.
7 Thakor NV, Webster JG. Electrode studies for the long-term ambulatory ECG. *Med Biol Eng Comput* 1985; **23**: 116–21.
8 Doss JD, McCabe CW, Weiss GK. Noise-free ECG data during electrosurgical procedures. *Anesth Analg* 1973; **52**: 156–60.
9 Ridley P. Implications of the Electromagnetic Compatibility Directive. *Electr Communicat Eng J* 1995, October: 195–9.
10 IEC 601–1 (EN60601–1, BS 5724, Pt. 1). *Medical electrical equipment. Part 1: General requirements for safety*. Geneva: International Electrotechnical Commission, 1988.
11 IEC 1000–4–2 (BS EN 61000–4–2). *Section 2: Electrostatic discharges. Immunity test*. Geneva International Electrotechnical Commission (in preparation).
12 IEC 1000–4–3 (BS EN 61000–4–3). *Section 3: Immunity to radiated RF electrical fields*. Geneva: International Electrotechnical Commission (in preparation).

13 Russell PH, Coakley CS. Electrocardiographic observation in the operating room. *Anesth Analg* 1969; **48**: 784–8.
14 Blackburn H, Katigbak R. What electrocardiographic leads to take after exercise? *Am Heart J* 1964; **67**: 184–5.
15 Pipberger HV, Arzbaecher RC, Berson AS. *et al.* Report of the committee on Electrocardiography, American Heart Association: Recommendations for standardization of leads and specification for instruments in electrocardiography and vectorcardiography. *Circulation* 1975; **52**: 11.
16 Bazarai MG, Norfleet EA. Comparison of CB_5 and V_5 leads for intraoperative electrocardiographic monitoring. *Anesth Analg* 1981; **60**: 849–53.
17 Burch CE. History of precordial leads in electrocardiography. *Eur J Cardiol* 1978; **8**: 207–36.
18 Kaplan JA, King SB. The precordial electrocardiographic lead (V_5) in patients who have coronary artery disease. *Anesthesiology* 1976; **45**: 570–4.
19 Froelicher VF, Wolthius R, Keiser N *et al.* A comparison of two bipolar exercise electrocardiographic leads to lead V5. *Chest* 1976; **70**: 611–16.
20 Kates RA, Zaidan JR, Kaplan JA. Esophageal lead for intraoperative electrocardiographic monitoring. *Anesth Analg* 1982; **61**: 781–5.
21 Greeley WJ, Kates RA, Bushman GA, Armstrong BE, Grant JW. Intraoperative esophageal electrocardiography for dysrhythmia analysis and therapy in pediatric cardiac surgical patients. *Anesthesiology* 1986; **65**: 669–72.
22 Lewes D. Electrode jelly in electrocardiography. *Br Heart J* 1965; **27**: 105–15.
23 IEC 601–2–25. *Particular requirements for the safety of electrocardiographs.* Geneva: International Electrotechnical Commission, 1993.
24 IEC 601–2–27. *Particular requirements for the safety of electrocardiographic monitoring equipment.* Geneva: International Electrotechnical Commission, 1994.
25 IEC 601–2–4. *Particular requirements for the safety of cardiac defibrillators and monitors.* Geneva: International Electrotechnical Commission (revision in preparation).
26 American Heart Association. Report of a committee on electrocardiography. *Circulation* 1967; **35**: 583–602.
27 Hull, CJ. The electrical hazards of patient monitoring. In: Hutton P, Prys-Roberts, C. *Monitoring in anaesthesia and intensive care.* London: W.B. Saunders Company Ltd, 1994: 56–77.
28 *The report of the expert working group on alarms on clinical monitors.* London: Medical Devices Agency, 1995: 11–23.
29 IEC 930. *Guidance for administrative, medical, and nursing staff concerned with the safe use of medical electrical equipment.* Geneva: International Electrotechnical Commission, 1988.
30 Health Equipment Information No. 98. *Management of medical equipment and devices.* Medical Devices Directorate. London: Department of Health, 1991.

3 Diagnostic scope and limitations of ECG monitoring

Medical

Hospital

The use of ECG monitoring in hospital departments of diagnostic cardiology and its specialist use in coronary care and cardiac surgical after-care units is beyond the scope of this book and the reader is referred to standard texts on the subject.

Nevertheless, it is a part of all doctors' training and experience to become familiar with such basic interpretation of the ECG as will enable them to differentiate between the grossly normal and abnormal. Similarly, nurses are increasingly acquainted with the bedside ECG and those who are experienced in coronary or intensive care may acquire a degree of competence. Moreover, as a result of the trend towards treating patients outside major institutions where this is feasible, general practitioners are being encouraged to expand their range of interests and expertise and many now appreciate the part they may play in the monitoring and diagnosis of patients with potential or actual cardiac problems. The role of paramedical staff now extends to the monitoring of patients at accident sites and in transit to or between medical installations. Thus, all who find themselves in such circumstances should equip themselves accordingly.

Individual expertise

In case those not immediately concerned in the institutional care of patients with abnormal ECGs think that hospital doctors are generally more competent in this respect, it is worth reflecting on the fact that several studies[1,2] have demonstrated the lack of competence of many hospital doctors in very basic interpretation of the ECG. It has also been shown that simple formal instruction and programmed learning can improve the diagnostic ability of individuals very rapidly.[2] It would therefore seem that, given the abundance of source material in textbooks, manuals, poster

41

material, audiovisual programmes, interactive computer learning, and formal courses, it is feasible for all with the requisite interest to attain a useful level of competence. There are several monographs on the subject.[3-6]

Automated interpretation

Automated interpretation is increasingly used in diagnostic cardiology. Instruments range from those concerned with a particular aspect of the ECG trace[7-9] to those offering fully automatic interpretation of the cardiac record; provision may be arranged beside the patient or more remotely. This approach is not new,[10] but the reliability of the implemented systems has often been suspect.[11] Expert systems have been devised and show promise[12] and neural networks have been invoked[8,9]. Some guidance is available[13] and the performance of some systems has been assessed.[14]

Anaesthesia and surgery

The basic physiology of the myocardial cell membrane in terms of its importance in anaesthesia has been reviewed by Merin,[15] and the place of the ECG in the monitoring of anaesthesia dealt with by several studies.[16-19]

The presence of a clinically satisfactory ECG trace does not necessarily confirm the adequacy of cardiac output. It was shown shortly after the general introduction of electrocardiography into monitoring during anaesthesia that, in animals at least, cessation of cardiac output might not be reflected in corresponding changes in the ECG for several minutes.[20] Indeed, whilst ECG changes indicating abnormalities of conduction of the electrical impulse may be relayed promptly, it must be remembered that deficiencies in the myocardium and its perfusion may be independent of the conducting system and only demonstrated when the conducting system itself is affected. The dangers associated with misinterpretation of the ECG when only a monitor trace is available should be borne in mind.[21,22]

The ECG trace may, however, provide the first intimation of a number of important complications during the course of anaesthesia. Examples which may be quoted are: arrythmias;[23,24] including those occurring during intubation;[25] during traction on ocular muscles and peritoneum;[26,27] during the administration of nitrous oxide;[28] and in myocardial ischaemia.[29-31] Other intraoperative cardiovascular abnormalities are detectable during anaesthesia,[32] and the mechanism of cardiac arryhthmias has been extensively reviewed.[33]

The detection of ischaemia before serious damage ensues is of especial concern to the anaesthetist. Several accounts have dealt with this aspect of anaesthetic monitoring.[34-39] The ECG has also been compared with transoesophageal echocardiography.[40,41]

The S-T segment has properly received special attention as that part of the ECG trace most likely to warn of ischaemia during anaesthesia,[42] and even neonates have been noted to provide such evidence.[43] The principle has been extended throughout the perioperative period,[44,45] and attempts have been made to analyse the immediate output by computer to determine which leads were most appropriate.[46] Nevertheless, the S-T segment is particularly susceptible to artefact as a result of movement or even of inadequate design of the instrument.[47] Changes in the R-wave may have special significance in cardiac surgery.[48] As has been noted in Chapter 2, the placement of electrodes[49] and the conditions under which traces and recordings are obtained may limit the confidence which may be placed in the observations.

Goldman proposed a number of cardiovascular risk factors in the production of morbidity in association with anaesthesia,[50,51] and Tarhan and colleagues have examined the risk of myocardial infarction in particular.[52] Preoperative ECG investigation is a logical consequence and may yield useful information concerning the propensity of patients to develop problems intraoperatively[39,53] or postoperatively.[38] Callaghan and colleagues note that the practice may, however, be abused,[54] and the value of the routine invocation of this and other preoperative investigations is questionable.[55-58] The detailed review by Mangano is especially valuable.[59] Ambulatory monitoring, although superficially attractive has proved disappointing.[60] A survey of the role and limitations of the ECG in connection with anaesthesia was undertaken in the course of a review of 2000 incidents in an Australian study.[61] Some patients may be especially susceptible to cardiac electrical stimulation.[62]

Dental anaesthesia is less prevalent than formerly, but may be conducted outside institutions which might be expected routinely to provide monitoring for local and general anaesthesia. Unfortunately, deaths and serious morbidity in the dental chair occur from time to time, sometimes affecting seemingly fit young subjects. It is especially important that, in circumstances where fitness may be assumed but not easily confirmed, and where operator and anaesthetist must control the airway whilst dental work is undertaken, appropriate monitoring, including the ECG, be established. Guidance may be found in the report of the Clinical Standards Advisory Group.[63]

Intensive care unit

Monitoring in the intensive care setting is often the responsibility of the nurse and may be undertaken at the bedside, centrally (at a monitoring station) or both. Whilst central monitoring[64] has proved popular in the detection of arrhythmias, when nurses are specifically involved,[65] automatic arrhythmia detection has had mixed success.[66] However, the relative

43

interdependence of different physiological systems, as seen in multiple system failure, has placed the principal burden on the bedside nurse. It is important that proper attention is given to the quality of the electrocardiographic monitoring information provided.[67–70]

General practice

The ECG can be a useful monitoring tool in general practice. Although the conditions in a busy surgery may not be those of the cardiac investigation unit, monitoring undertaken with suitable equipment in the consulting room of the surgery can yield sufficiently faithful traces and records to indicate obvious arrhythmias and ischaemia. Despite the pressures of time during general practice consultation, it is nevertheless just as important that proper preparation of the electrode sites is undertaken, that the electrodes are satisfactorily placed and secured, and that the patient is given time to relax and adjust to the circumstances of the monitoring session.

Unless the practitioner is experienced in the immediate interpretation of the ECG, it is prudent to obtain a hard-copy record of the session or pertinent parts of it for examination later or for consideration by a colleague with greater experience. One of the benefits of monitoring, as opposed to "spot" recordings, is that the record can be examined for consistency and for the recurrence of transient phenomena.

Stress testing is potentially hazardous and best undertaken by practitioners with special training and experience or under the supervision of a cardiologist.

Domiciliary

There are also attractions in being able to transfer the monitoring session to the patient's own home. With the emergence of highly competent practice nurses, it would seem not unreasonable to take the opportunity of obtaining ECG monitoring records under the congenial conditions of the home in the presence of a familiar nurse. A number of rugged, compact units are available. The precautions already alluded to are equally mandatory. In addition, there is a special need to make sure that the ECG equipment used is in good condition and well maintained, that it is suitable for transport and domiciliary use and that its users are properly trained.

44

Emergency

The emergency use of ECG monitoring falls into three distinct categories: in the accident and emergency unit, the ward emergency and emergencies elsewhere.

Accident and Emergency unit

The quality of ECG monitoring in Accident & Emergency departments has improved dramatically with the establishment of specialist consultant posts in the speciality and the consequently improved quality and training of students in the discipline. Whilst it is appropriate to summon cardiological staff to carry out 12-lead diagnostic ECGs when these are indicated, the place of ECG monitoring instituted by the A&E staff themselves should not be overlooked. Most medical staff working long term in the A&E department expect to acquire a good deal of general diagnostic and therapeutic experience. One of the commonest presentations is the patient with chest pain, giddiness or some other possible manifestation of acute cardiovascular disease. The benefit of monitoring in this setting is that obvious abnormalities of rhythm and frank ischaemia may be recognised quickly and dealt with. Moreover, continued monitoring provides the opportunity to assess the immediate progress of the patient and any significant trends. Hard-copy records can be taken at any point and facilities now exist for the output to be electronically transmitted to experts for an opinion or comparison with existing records. However, the ECG may sometimes be misleading.[71] For example, in one study it was found that 3% of patients who had sustained a myocardial infarction had a normal ECG, whilst a further 7% had non-specific ECG changes only.[72,73] The benefits generally outweigh such disadvantages, but it is clearly important, in addition to appraising the ECG trace, to exercise prudent clinical judgement based on associated findings. It has been suggested that a normal ECG virtually excludes cardiac failure in emergency patients in whom it is suspected.[74]

The ward emergency

The position of ECG monitoring in the ward setting is less satisfactory. It is uncommon for medical staff to take a direct interest in the ECG monitoring of patients who are not under the direct supervision of cardiologists or physicians with a cardiological interest. The task is therefore, more often than not, delegated to nurses who may or may not have any experience with the ECG. It is a matter for concern that this particular form of monitoring, though perhaps less glamorous than certain other forms of monitoring and treatment, is accorded less than due respect. This is certainly true when patients are admitted as emergencies to general wards, but also occurs when patients are considered by their medical advisors to need ECG monitoring selectively and have this prescribed without further advice or instruction. Whether the benefits of ECG monitoring in general wards match its widespread use in this manner is uncertain.

Emergencies elsewhere

The emergency use of ECG monitoring in circumstances other than those described may be disparate, yet it is often undertaken by enthusiastic general practitioners, who may be members of designated emergency teams and by mobile squads attending accidents and disasters. Some excellent equipment is currently available for ECG monitoring in such circumstances. Devices are rugged, may have LCD or plasma displays, are light and compact, battery or mains operated and may, in some cases, be placed directly on the precordium. Even these small instruments can provide hardcopy output. As always, it is essential that the observer has experience sufficient to assure sensible interpretation of the trace obtained, with some appreciation of the possible pitfalls. For example, a flat trace obtained under these conditions may not necessarily reflect cardiac arrest, but could represent an unsatisfactory trace of, for example, ventricular fibrillation.[75]

Nursing

Hospital

Although the inappropriate delegation of ECG monitoring to untrained or insufficiently trained nurses is to be deprecated, more nurses are undertaking specialist nurse practitioner training. They may be expected to become highly skilled in the manner of the nurses who so effectively staff intensive therapy and coronary care units. The prevalence of ECG monitoring in non-cardiac wards suggests that this element of training should enjoy a high priority.

Community

The change in emphasis prompted by the NHS reforms, such that more treatment is likely to take place outside hospital than formerly, has thrown an unexpectedly large burden on those providing care in the community. Those, other than general practitioners, most concerned with the patients' medical care and, indeed, usually providing continuity of care, are for the

46

most part community nurses, whose training, skill and experience renders them able and adaptable. Early discharge of patients from hospital and devolution of certain types of treatment from hospital to the home make it likely that some forms of monitoring, formerly the exclusive preserve of the hospital, may legitimately be undertaken in the home. Should this prove to be the case, the supervision of such patients, although the ultimate responsibility of the general practitioner, might well fall to the community nurse. There seems no obvious reason why community nurses should not be effective in this role, provided appropriate training is given. The possibility of relaying the output of ECG monitors and recorders to remote sites for interpretation is perhaps comparable with domiciliary obstetric monitoring undertaken during pregnancy with considerable success by midwives, community nurses and often the patients themselves.

Specific aspects of ECG monitoring

The foregoing has been concerned largely with ECG monitoring as an episodic undertaking in a static environment. However, the general usefulness of the technique inside and outside conventional care institutions merits further consideration.

Trend appreciation

Whilst examination of the ECG for diagnostic purposes is widely practised in a variety of disciplines and settings, its use as a trend analyser has become widespread during the past 20 years or so. It is therefore used in hospitals and clinics, for cardiac assessment during exercise or stress testing,[76–78] in clinics for the assessment of change over a period of time, and for screening in community clinics, private health clinics and in industry. Moreover, there is a potential to realise the benefits of real-time analysis.[79]

Stress testing

Stress testing enjoys justifiable popularity as a means of determining threshold for ischaemia and the onset of significant arrhythmias. However, it is not without its dangers and certain precautions need to be taken in its use.[80–82]

ECG telemetry

Remote on-line monitoring of patients has become possible following the successful transmission of medical signals such as the ECG recorded in the hospital ward or out-patient clinic, in the general practitioner's consulting room or in the patient's home,[83,84] over increasing distances, thanks to advances in telecommunications.[85-87] Fetal ECGs may be transmitted similarly.[88] Not only may simple, single-channel ECG trace information be transmitted, but more complex multiple-channel information, perhaps accompanied by other physiological data and images, is increasingly feasible. A good review is that of McClelland *et al.*[89] Alternatively, hard-copy obtained from monitoring traces recorded remotely and/or transmitted by radio or telephone may be analysed at leisure by experts.

The transmission of patient data via local or wider networks, and over national and international telecommunications systems, raises issues of concern in respect of patient confidentiality. This is especially true in the use of the virtually uncontrolled Internet. However, the provision in several countries of national communications networks partly or wholly dedicated to health care may help overcome some of the genuine anxieties concerning the integrity, security and privacy of the transmitted data. In Europe, European Standards (CEN) Technical Committee 251 is tackling a number of the problems concerning standardisation of the formats in which data of this kind should be transmitted electronically. Its Working Group 5 has already produced a document dealing with the transmission of analysed electrocardiographic data[90] and Working Group 6 is concerned with data security.

Ambulatory ECG monitoring

An interesting and rewarding application of ECG monitoring has been the ambulatory monitoring of subjects as they go about their normal daily activities and sometimes also through the sleeping hours.[91] It has a particular place in monitoring the elderly without immobilisation and its attendant risks,[92] although its predictive value has been disputed.[93] Criteria for suitable equipment have been established.[94]

1 Montgomery H, Hunter S, Morris S, Naunton-Morgan R, Marshall RM. Interpretation of electrocardiograms by doctors. *BMJ* 1994; **309**: 1551–2.
2 Woodmansey PA, White TA, Channer KS. Formal teaching can reduce serious errors in interpretation. *BMJ* 1995; **310**: 468.
3 Fleming JS. *Interpreting the electrocardiogram*. London: Update Books, 1979.
4 Davis D. *How to quickly and accurately master ECG interpretation*. Philadelphia: JB Lippincott Co, 1985.
5 Atlee JJ III. Perioperative Cardiac Dysrhythmias, 2nd edn. Chicago: Year Book, 1990.

6 Bennett DH. *Cardiac arrhythmias. Practical notes on interpretation and treatment.* 4th edn. Oxford: Butterworth Heinemann, 1993.

7 Burns MP, Downs WG. Clinical evaluation of a bedside ST-segment monitor. *IEEE Comput Cardiol* 1988; **97**: 100.

8 Edenbrandt L, Devine B, Macfarlane PW. Neural networks for classification of ECG ST-T segments. *J Electrocardiol* 1992; **25**: 167–73.

9 Suzuki Y, Ono K. Personal computer system for ECG ST-segment recognition based on neural networks. *Med Biol Eng Comput* 1992; **30**: 2–8.

10 Caceres C, Hochberg HM. Performance of the computer and physician in the analysis of the electrocardiogram. *Am Heart J* 1970; **79**: 439–43.

11 Editorial. How reliable is the computerized electrocardiographic interpretation? *JAMA* 1975; **231**: 1090.

12 Ong K, Chia P, Choo M. Real-time expert system for ECG diagnosis. *Proc Wld Cong Expert Systems*, Portugal, January 1994.

13 Pipberger HV, Cornfeld J. What ECG-computer program to choose for clinical application: the need for consumer protection. *Circulation* 1973; **47**: 918–20.

14 Willems JL, Abreu-Lima C, Arnaud P, *et al.* The diagnostic performance of computer programs for the interpretation of electrocardiograms. *N Engl J Med* 1991; **325**: 1767–73.

15 Merin RG. Cardiac cell membrane physiology: implications for the anaesthesiologist. *Curr Opinion Anaesthesiol* 1995; **8**: 1–6.

16 Thys DM, Kaplan JA eds. *The ECG in anesthesia and critical care.* New York: Churchill Livingstone, 1987.

17 Tyers MR, Russell WJ, Runciman WB. Electrocardiographic monitoring in anaesthesia. *Anaesth Intens Care* 1988; **16**: 66–9.

18 Weinfurt PT. Electrocardiographic monitoring: an overview. *J Clin Monit* 1990: **6**; 132–8.

19 Narang J, Thys DM. Electrocardiographic monitoring. In Ehrenwerth J, Eisenkraft JB eds. *Anesthesia equipment: principles and applications.* St. Louis: Mosby, 1993.

20 Mazzia VDB, Ellis CH, Siegel H, Hershey SG. The electrocardiograph as a monitor of cardiac function in the operating room. *JAMA* 1966; **198**: 103–7.

21 Arbeit SR, Rubin IL, Gross H. Dangers in interpreting the electrocardiogram from the oscilloscope monitor. *JAMA* 1970; **211**: 453–6.

22 Brock PJM, Bowes JB. Forum: Limitations of electrocardioscopy – failure of the electrocardiograph to warn of low cardiac output. *Anaesthesia* 1975; **30**: 90–4.

23 Dodd RB, Sims WA, Bone DJ. Cardiac arrhythmias observed during anesthesia. *Surgery* 1962; **51**: 440.

24 Kuner J, Enescu V, Utsu F, Boszormenyi E, Bernstein H, Corday E. Cardiac arrhythmias during anaesthesia. *Dis Chest* 1967; **52**: 580–7.

25 Bertrand CA, Steiner NV, Jamieson AG, Lopez M. Disturbances of cardiac rhythm during anesthesia and surgery. *JAMA* 1971; **216**: 1615–17.

26 Deacock AR de C, Oxer HF. The prevention of reflex bradycardia during ophthalmic surgery. *Brit J Anaesth* 1962; **34**: 451–7.

27 Coventry DM, McMenemin I, Lawrie S. Bradycardia during abdominal surgery – modification by pre-operative cholinergic agents. *Anaesthesia* 1987; **42**: 835–9.

28 Roizen MF, Plummer GO, Lichter JL. Nitrous oxide and dysrhythmias. *Anesthesiology* 1987; **66**: 427–30.

29 De Hert SG, De Jongh RF, Van den Bossche AO, De Maere PL, Adriaensen HF. The detection of intraoperative myocardial ischaemia. *Anaesthesia* 1989; **44**: 881–4.

30 Slogoff S, Keats AS. Does perioperative myocardial ischaemia lead to postoperative myocardial infarction? *Anesthesiology* 1985; **62**: 107–14.

31 Griffin RN, Kaplan JA. Intraoperative myocardial ischaemia. In: Thys DM, Kaplan JA, eds. *The ECG in anesthesia and critical care.* New York: Churchill Livingstone, 1987.

32 Stokes DN, Davies MK. Monitoring the electrical activity of the heart. In: Hutton P, Prys-Roberts C, eds. *Monitoring in anaesthesia and intensive care.* Oxford: Blackwell, 1994.

33 Atlee JL, Bosniak ZJ. Mechanism for cardiac dysrhythmias during anesthesia. *Anesthesiology* 1990; **72**: 347–74.

34 Raby KE, Barry J, Creager MA, Cook EF, Wisberg MC, Goldman L. Detection and significance of intraoperative and postoperative myocardial ischemia in peripheral vascular surgery. *JAMA* 1992; **268**: 222–7.

35 Kotrly KJ, Kotter GS, Mortara D, Kampaine JP. Intraoperative detection of myocardial ischemia with an ST segment trend montoring system. *Anesth Analg* 1984; **63**: 343–5.

36 Roy WL, Edelist G, Gilbert B. Myocardial ischemia during non-cardiac surgical procedures in patients with coronary artery disease. *Anesthesiology* 1979; **51**: 393–7.

37 Thomson IR, Rosenbloom M, Cannon JE, Morris M. Electrocardiographic S-T segment elevation after myocardial infarction during coronary artery surgery. *Anesth Analg* 1987; **66**: 1183–6.

38 London MJ, Hollenberg M, Wong MG *et al.* Intra-operative myocardial ischemia: localization by continuous 12-lead electrocardiography. *Anesthesiology* 1988; **69**: 232–41.

39 Fleischer LA, Rosenbaum SH, Nelson AH, Jain D, Wackers FJ, Zaret BL. Preoperative dipyridamole thallium imaging and ambulatory electrocardiographic monitoring as a predictor of perioperative cardiac events and long-term outcome. *Anesthesiology* 1995; **83**: 906–17.

40 Smith JS, Cahalan MK, Benefiel DJ *et al.* Intraoperative detection of myocardial ischemia in high-risk patients: electrocardiography versus two-dimensional transesophageal echocardiography. *Circulation* 1985; **72**: 1015–21.

41 Eisenberg MJ, London MJ, Leung JM, *et al.* Monitoring for myocardial ischemia during non-cardiac surgery. A technology assessment of transesophageal echocardiography and 12-lead electrocardiography. *JAMA* 1992; **268**: 210–16.

42 Foëx P, Prys-Roberts C. Anaesthesia and the hypertensive patient. *Brit J Anaesth* 1974; **46**: 575–88.

43 Bell C, Rimar S, Barash, P. Intraoperative S-T segment changes consistent with myocardial ischemia in the neonate: a report of three cases. *Anesthesiology* 1989; **71**: 601–4.

44 Griffin RM, Phipps JA, Evans JM. Electrocardiographical changes in the perioperative period. A pilot study. *Anaesthesia* 1985; **40**: 193–7.

45 Dodds TM, Delphin E, Stone G, Gal SG, Coromilas J. Detection of perioperative myocardial ischemia using Holter with real-time S-T segment analysis. *Anesth Analg* 1988; **67**: 890–3.

46 Griffin RN, Kaplan JA. Comparison of ECG V_5, CS_5, CB_5 and II by computerized ST segment analysis. *Anesth Analg* 1986; **65**: S1.

47 Tayler DI, Vincent R. Artefactual ST segment abnormalities due to electrocardiograph design. *Brit Heart J* 1985; **54**: 121–8.

48 Mark JB, Chien GL, Steinbrook RA, Fenton T. Electrocardiographic R-wave changes during cardiac surgery. *Anesth Analg* 1992; **74**: 26–31.

49 Kirstner JR, Miller ED, Epstein RM. More than V_5 needed. *Anesthesiology* 1977; **47**: 75–6.

50 Goldman L, Caldera DL, Nussbaum SR *et al.* Multifactorial index of cardiac risk in noncardiac surgical procedures. *New Engl J Med* 1977; **297**: 845–50.

51 Goldman L, Caldera DL, Southwick FS, Nussbaum SR, Murray B. Cardiac risk factors and complications in non-cardiac surgery. *Medicine* 1978; **57**: 357–70.

52 Tarhan S, Moffitt E, Taylor WF, Giulliani ER. Myocardial infarction after general anesthesia. *JAMA* 1972; **220**: 1451–4.

53 Mangano DT. Perioperative cardiac morbidity. *Anesthesiology* 1990; **72**: 153–84.

54 Callaghan LC, Edwards ND, Reilly CS. Utilisation of the preoperative ECG. *Anaesthesia* 1995; **50**: 488–90.

55 Patterson KR, Caskie JP, Galloway DL, McArthur K, McWhinnie DL. The pre-operative electrocardiogram: an assessment. *Scot Med J* 1983; **28**: 116–18.

56 Rabkin SW, Horne JM. Preoperative electrocardiography: effect of abnormalities on clinical decisions. *Can Med Ass J* 1983; **128**: 146–7.

57 Goldberger AL, O'Konski M. Utility of the routine electrocardiogram before surgery and on general hospital admission. *Ann Intern Med* 1986; **105**: 552–7.

58 McKee RF, Scott EM. The value of routine preoperative investigations. *Ann Roy Coll Surg* 1987; **69**: 160–2.

59 Mangano DT. Preoperative risk assessment: many studies, few solutions. Is a cardiac risk paradigm possible? *Anesthesiology* 1995; **83**: 897–901.

60 Raby KE, Goldman L, Creager MA, Cook EF *et al.* Correlation between preoperative ischemia and major cardiac events after peripheral vascular surgery. *N Engl J Med* 1989; **321**: 1296–300.

61 Ludbrook GL, Russell WJ, Webb RK, Klepper ID, Currie M. The electrocardiograph: applications and limitations – an analysis of 2000 incident reports. *Anaesth Intens Care* 1993; **21**: 558–64.

62 Leeming MN. Protection of the "electrically susceptible patient". *Anesthesiology* 1973; **38**: 370–83.

63 Clinical Standards Advisory Group. *Dental general anaesthesia*. London: HMSO, 1995.

64 Shah PM, Arnold JM, Haberern NA, Bliss DT, McClelland KM, Clarke WB. Automatic real-time arrhythmia monitoring in the intensive coronary care unit. *Am J Cardiol* 1977; **39**: 701–8.

65 Holmberg S, Ryder L, Waldenstrom A. Efficiency of arrhythmia detection by nurses in a coronary unit using a decentralized monitoring system. *Brit Heart J* 1977; **39**: 1019–22.

66 Romhilt DW, Bloomfield SS, Chou TC, Fowler NO. Unreliability of conventional electrocardiographic arrhythmia detection in coronary care unit. *Am J Cardiol* 1973; **31**: 457–61.

67 Runciman WB. Cardiovascular monitoring. *Crit Care Med* 1984; **3**: 2–3.

68 Griffin RN, Kaplan JA. ECG lead systems. In: Thys DM, Kaplan JA eds. *The ECG in anesthesia and critical care*. New York: Churchill Livingstone, 1987.

69 Gardner R.M, Hollingsworth KW. Optimizing the electrocardiogram and pressure monitoring. *Crit Care Med* 1986; **14**: 651–8.

70 Mirvis DM, Berson AS, Goldberger AL, *et al*. Instrumentation and practice standards for electrocardiographic monitoring in special care units. A report for health professionals by a Task Force of the Council on Clinical Cardiology, American Heart Association. *Circulation* 1989; **79**: 464–71.

71 Hedges JR, Kobernick MS. Detection of myocardial ischemia/infarction in the emergency department patient with chest discomfort. *Emerg Med Clin N Amer* 1988; **6**: 317–40.

72 Hedges JR. Pitfalls in accident and emergency pain evaluation. *J Roy Soc Med* 1995; **88**: 524–7P.

73 Field DL, Hedges JR, Arnold KJ, Goldstein-Wayne B, Rouan GW. Limitations of chest pain follow-up from an urban teaching hospital emergency department. *J Emerg Med* 1987; **6**: 636–8.

74 Davie AP, Francis CM, Love MP *et al*. Value of the electrocardiogram in identifying heart failure due to left ventricular systolic dysfunction. *BMJ* 1996; **312**: 222.

75 Cummins RO, Austin D Jr. The frequency of "occult" ventricular fibrillation masquerading as a flat line in prehospital cardiac arrest. *Ann Emerg Med* 1988; **17**: 813–17.

76 Fortuin NJ, Freisinger GC. Exercise-induced S-T segment elevation. *Am J Med* 1970; **49**: 459–64.

77 Hegge FN, Tuna N, Burchell HB. Coronary arteriographic findings in patients with axis shifts or S-T segment elevations on exercise-stress testing. *Am Heart J* 1973; **86**: 603–15.

78 Bonoris PE, Greenberg PS, Christison GW, Castellanet MJ, Ellestad MH. Evaluation of R amplitude changes versus S-T segment depression in stress testing. *Circulation* 1978; **57**: 904–10.

79 Levin RI, Cohen D, Frisbie W. Potential for real-time processing of the continuously monitored electrocardiogram in the detection, quantitation, and intervention of silent cardiac ischemia. *Cardiol Clin* 1986; **4**: 735–45.

80 Chaitman BR, Hanson JS. Comparative sensitivity and specificity of exercise electrocardiographic lead systems. *Am J Cardiol* 1981; **47**: 1335–49.

81 Mason RE, Likar IA. A new system of multiple-lead exercise electrocardiography. *Amer Heart J* 1966; **71**: 196–205.

82 Robertson D, Kostuk WJ, Ahuja SP. The localization of coronary artery stenoses by 12-lead ECG response to graded exercise test: support for coronary steal. *Am Heart J* 1976; **91**: 437–44.

83 Ong K, Chia P, Ng WL, Choo M. A telemedicine system for high-quality transmission of paper electrocardiographic reports. *J Telemed Telecare* 1995; **1**: 27–33.

84 Thorborg S, Sjoqvist BA. Mobimed – a telesystem for mobile monitoring of physiological parameters. *IEE, SPIE* 1990; (**1355**): 32–5.

85 Grigoriev AI, Egorov AD. Medical monitoring in long-term space missions: theory and experience. *Proc 43rd Congr Int Astronaut Fed*, Washington, September 1992.

86 Raymond CA. When medical help really is far away. *JAMA* 1988; **259**: 2343–4.

51

87 Chia P, Ong K, Choo M. Real-time compression and detection of ECG signals. *Proc Seventh Int Congr Biomed Eng*, Singapore, December 1992.

88 Fisk NM, Bower S, Seulveda W *et al*. Fetal telemedicine: interactive transfer of realtime ultrasound and video via ISDN for remote consultation. *J Telemed Telecare* 1995; **1**: 38–44.

89 McClelland I, Adamson K, Black ND. Information issues in telemedicine systems. *J Telemed Telecare* 1995; **1**: 7–12.

90 *ENV 1064. Medical informatics – Standard communication protocol – Computer assisted cardiography.* Brussels: European Committee for Standardisation (CEN), 1993.

91 Morganroth J. Ambulatory Holter electrocardiography: choice of technique and clinical uses. *Ann Intern Med* 1985; **102**: 73–81.

92 Raiha IJ, Piha SJ, Seppanen P, Puukka P, Sourander LB. Predictive value of continuous ambulatory cardiographic monitoring in elderly people. *BMJ* 1994; **309**: 1263–7.

93 Bassan M Continuous ambulatory electrocardiography in elderly people. *BMJ* 1995; **310**: 468.

94 Sheffield LT, Berson AS, Bragg-Remschel D *et al*. Recommendations for standards of instrumentation and practice in the use of ambulatory electrocardiography. The task force committee on electrocardiography and cardiac electrophysiology of the council on clinical cardiology. *Circulation* 1985; **71**: 626–36A.

4 Non-invasive blood pressure (NIBP) monitoring

Historical outline

The earliest attempts to measure blood pressure were undertaken in animals, using cannulation of blood vessels for direct measurements. It was not until the close of the nineteenth century that successful indirect means were achieved.

Much earlier, William Harvey, in his *De motu cordis*,[1,2] published in 1628, described the manner in which the heart moved. Harvey concluded that that the blood circulated within the body and that the heart was responsible for maintaining the flow by its pumping action.

Hales – experiments with the horse

The measurement of blood pressure may be traced back to 1733, when the Reverend Stephen Hales placed a tube in the femoral artery of a horse. He noted that the height of the column of blood in the tube rose to more than 8 ft.[3,4] Moreover, the column of blood rose and fell in time with the pulse and there appeared to be a variation related to the horse's pattern of breathing.

There appear to have been no more significant developments until 1828, when Poiseuille used a U-tube containing mercury for the measurement of blood pressure in the dog.[5]

Vierordt – counter pressure

In 1854, Vierordt devised an apparatus based on the pressure required to occlude a blood vessel and cause the cessation of pulsation in it.[4] His sphygmograph was large and heavy and does not appear to have achieved popularity.

Faivre – using Poiseuille's manometer

Faivre described the application of Poiseuille's technique to the severed limb arteries of amputees. Again, oscillations corresponding with the pulse were observed, as was the fact that there was a small variation with breathing.[4,6] Thus, what we would now recognise as the *mean* arterial blood pressure was determined.

Marey – mercury-filled tube and pressure cuff

It was not until twenty years later that Marey, improving upon Vierordt's sphygmograph, described a technique in which the forearm was occluded by the pressure of a circumferential cuff until blanching occurred.[4,7] The pressure in the cuff was transmitted to a mechanical recorder, yielding what was the forerunner of much of today's indirect measurement apparatus. Potain[4] observed that the characteristics of the arterial wall could affect the performance of the instrument. Marey's sphygmograph was further improved by Dudgeon[4] and by Von Basch[8,9] who, with Zadek, had noted that patients with hardened arteries had higher blood pressures than most subjects.

The Riva-Rocci apparatus

An improved pneumatic cuff was introduced by Riva-Rocci in 1896, in conjunction with a mercury-filled manometer tube (Figure 4.1).[9] The pressure in the cuff could be correlated with the reappearance of a pulse at the wrist when the cuff was applied to the upper arm. Riva-Rocci's cuff was 5 cm wide.

A flurry of improvements appeared in the next few years. First, Hill and Barnard (1897)[10] elaborated the Riva-Rocci method, furnishing their instrument with a dial pressure gauge. Shortly afterwards, von Recklinghausen drew attention to the need for the cuff size to be commensurate with that of the limb from which measurements were being taken (1901),[11,12] recommending a cuff of 12 cm width for the arm. Korotkoff[13] described his well-known sounds in 1905.[14] Korotkoff was also responsible for the binaural stethoscope subsequently used in the technique.[15] It was proposed by Codman and Cushing[16] that the blood pressure be measured routinely during surgery and at clinic visits but, although we may regard this as the beginnings of blood pressure monitoring in the operating theatre and of routine blood pressure screening in the out-patient clinic and practice consulting room, it appears that it was not well received in the authors' institution. Nevertheless, blood pressure

54

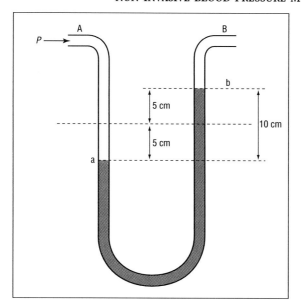

Figure 4.1(a) A simple U-tube manometer is filled with water. When pressure is applied to limb A the fluid in limb A is depressed and that in B raised. The difference between the levels at A and B indicates the pressure applied, in this case 10 cm of water.[D]

measurement was of sufficient general medical interest for textbooks on the subject to appear in the USA and Europe.[17,18]

Recordings were crude at that time and could not reflect the frequency-dependent components of recorded waveforms faithfully. The kymograph had been introduced by Ludwig in 1847,[19] and, at the turn of the century Frank introduced an optical recording system capable of responding to these components and correctly reproducing the peaks and the dicrotic notch of blood pressure waveforms. More refined optical systems followed, but have since been joined by electronic writing devices and visual displays.[20]

What is the blood pressure?

The blood perfusing the body by way of the arteries does so in a pulsatile manner as the result of the pumping action of the heart. With each cardiac contraction, blood is driven into the aorta against the resistance of the system into which it is ejecting the blood, i.e. the *systemic vascular resistance* (SVR). This may be expressed in the form: *pressure = flow × resistance*. The flow is effectively the cardiac output (CO).

The blood flows from the left ventricle, through the open aortic valve, into the aorta which, being distensible and elastic, expands to accommodate

55

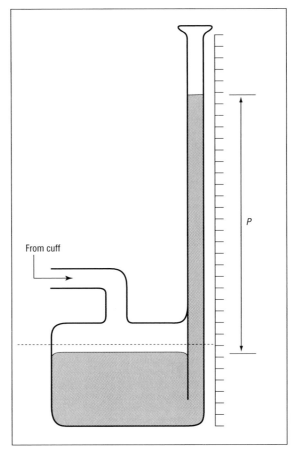

Figure 4.1(b) Illustrating the principle of the mercury sphygmomanometer, the pressure in the cuff is applied to the surface of a pool of mercury. Since this forms what is, in effect, a large bore limb of a U-tube, only a small displacement of the mercury level takes place compared with that in the narrow vertical limb (to the right) which is calibrated in terms of the pressure P to be measured. The calibration approximates the height of the mercury in this limb alone.[D]

the extra blood. It further allows its passage and adjusts its calibre to the pattern of flow during ejection.

When maximum ejection from the left ventricle into the aorta is taking place, i.e. during systole, it may be expected that the pressure required to overcome the resistance to flow will be at a maximum. Thus we may establish that the *systolic pressure* is the maximum pressure generated during cardiac ejection into the vascular outflow when measured at some point in that outflow.

As the blood passes through the arterial system during systole, it encounters resistance in the more peripheral vessels which, by reason of their elasticity and vascular tone, maintain flow at the levels needed in

---

Blood pressure

Systolic pressure
The maximum pressure in the main arteries resulting from the ejection of blood from the left ventricle.

Diastolic pressure
The pressure in the main arteries when cardiac ejection has ceased.

Pulse pressure
The difference between the systolic and diastolic pressures.

Mean pressure (MAP)
May be expressed as: cardiac output (CO) × systemic vascular resistance (SVR).

---

various parts of the body. Thus, it is possible to estimate the blood pressure at points beyond that at which it is ejected from the heart and the accessibility of an artery will generally dictate its usefulness as a site for the measurement of the blood pressure. However, the shape of the waveform representing the changes in pressure during the cardiac cycle varies at different points in the peripheral circulation (Figure 4.2). This is due in part to the changing calibre of the vessels as they pass peripherally and in part to the fact that, when blood has been pumped to the periphery, there is a small rebound effect in the distensible system which, as it were, drives the blood back into the face of the next ejection of blood from the heart, marginally adding to the pressure generated. The *dicrotic notch* of the blood pressure waveform is one result of this phenomenon (Figure 4.3).

The effect is more marked in subjects whose blood vessels are dilated and less marked in those whose vessels are constricted. A further consequence of this is that the pressures measured in the radial artery at the wrist, the brachial artery at the elbow and the femoral artery at the groin differ accordingly (Figure 4.4).

As each left ventricular ejection is completed, the energy imparted to the blood leaving the heart falls towards zero, so that the pressure in the aorta during diastole is that maintained by the SVR. Back flow is prevented by closure of the aortic valve, but the elasticity in the peripheral arteries imparts some backwards-directed energy to the blood in the aorta, yielding a transient rise in pressure before an equilibrium is reached between the pressure of the blood and the elastic and tonic effect of the containing blood vessels. At this point, no appreciable change in pressure occurs and the position is maintained until the left ventricle once again contracts and forces the blood in it past the opening aortic valve into the aorta. The pressure at which the blood pressure is maintained at the low equilibrium level is the *diastolic pressure*. In the absence of cardiac output during diastole,

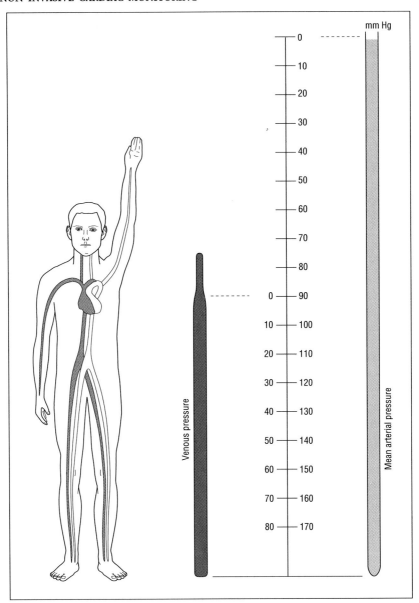

Figure 4.2 Mean arterial pressure in the upright posture. The venous pressure behaves in a similar manner.[E]

it is principally dependent upon the systemic vascular resistance. An important corollary is that pressure of itself is an inadequate indicator of perfusion and is of limited value unless some knowledge of cardiac output and systemic vascular resistance is available, however crudely. The

58

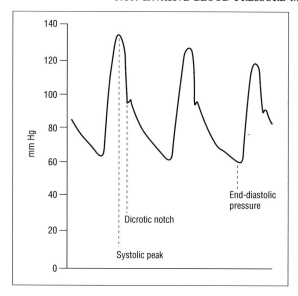

Figure 4.3 The arterial pressure waveform, showing the dicrotic notch.[E]

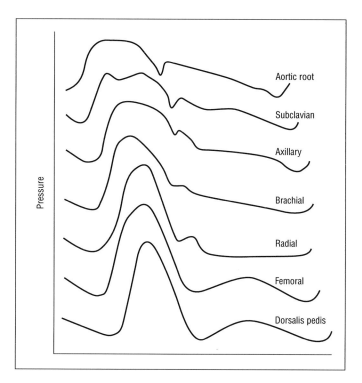

Figure 4.4 Configuration of the pressure-pulse wave at various sites in the arterial tree.[F]

difference between the systolic and diastolic pressures is the *pulse pressure* which, in a limited way, reflects the stroke volume ejected during systole. Despite the influence of other variables, change in the pulse pressure is in many circumstances a useful indicator of changes in the stroke volume. It has also been shown that, on account of the decrease in vascular calibre and the associated increase in the velocity of the blood, the pulse pressure increases with the distance from the heart.[21]

The *mean pressure* represents the effective perfusion pressure. Since it is dependent upon cardiac output (CO) and the systemic vascular resistance (SVR), mean arterial pressure (MAP) equates to $CO \times SVR$. An approximation to the mean arterial pressure may be achieved by use of the following equation:

$$MAP = \frac{systolic + (diastolic \times 2)}{3}$$

In practice, the SVR cannot be measured directly. A useful approximation may be derived by use of the following formula:

$$SVR = \frac{MAP}{CO} \times 80 \ (normal \ value = 900 - 1400 \ dynes/s/cm^{-5})$$

Another method of deriving the mean pressure is based on the area under the waveform curve. The computation of the area was formerly achieved by planimetry, but the production by microprocessor-based devices of series of digital values representing points on the curve nowadays permits automatic calculation.

Posture is a major determinant of perfusion in different parts of the body. It is assumed that pressures throughout the body are similar when the subject is recumbent, but this is certainly not the case when the subject is erect. Figure 4.2 shows the approximate MAP in a normal adult in the upright posture, where it can be seen that MAP varies from some 40 mm Hg in the elevated hand to more than 170 mm Hg in the foot. It should be noted especially that the perfusion pressure presented to the brain is substantially less than that at the level of the heart.

The term "blood pressure" is generally understood to refer to the relationship between the systolic and diastolic pressures and is conventionally expressed as, for example 130/80, the units being millimetres of mercury. Most medical measurement values should be stated in Système Internationale (SI) units, but certain permitted measurements have been declared. In this instance, in addition to the SI unit of kilopascals (kPa), the mm Hg is a permitted unit for blood pressure, a unit hallowed by convention and use and thus very familiar.

Although the pair of values is often quoted as the "normal" adult value, it is more properly expressed as a range of such values. It is important to

60

Typical values for paediatric blood pressure*

- Adult: 130/80 mm Hg (systolic range 100–140 mm Hg)
- Adolescent (15 years): 110–130 mm Hg
- Schoolchild (7 years): 95–110 mm Hg systolic
- Child of 2 years: 95–105 mm Hg systolic
- Neonate/small infant: 85–105 mm Hg systolic

* Based on Horan, MJ *Pediatrics* 1987; **79**:1

---

remember that children have blood pressure values in a lower range, whilst neonates and small infants may have systolic pressure of only 75–85 mm Hg.

It is not our purpose here to argue the case for different pressure levels in the definition of hypertension, nor to pursue the maladies associated with disturbances of blood pressure, but to define what it is we intend to measure and then to demonstrate the indirect (i.e. non-invasive) means of doing that.

Methods of measurement of blood pressure

Palpation

Simple palpation of a peripheral pulse may be used to establish that the pulse has returned during reduction of the pressure in an occluding limb cuff. Similarly, the disappearance of the pulse is used to determine the point at which the cuff pressure exceeds that in the occluded artery.

It has been shown that the method is influenced by the rate of the heart and, more especially, by the rate of deflation of the cuff, and that the directly measured systolic pressure is generally underestimated. Van Bergen et al.[22] showed the extent of this underestimation as being some 30 mm Hg at a directly measured systolic pressure of 120 mm Hg (Figure 4.5).

As a rough and ready means of establishing the approximate level of the systolic pressure, however, the method has much to commend it, since no additional equipment is required. It is sometimes stated that if the radial pulse can be felt, the systolic blood pressure must be at least 80 mm Hg. However, in conditions in which vasodilatation is a feature, this may not be so, although the reduction in SVR may well be promoting better perfusion at the prevailing pressure than would normally be the case.

Palpating the pulse at the wrist is performed with the palpator placed comfortably, preferably sitting, with the seated subject's arm extended sufficiently to bring the wrist close to the level of the heart. The pulse is detected by the palmar tips of the middle or ring fingers, the wrist being

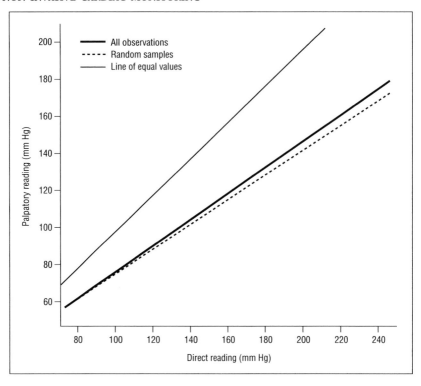

*Figure 4.5 Comparison of palpatory with direct blood pressure recordings;[1] and Van Bergen et al., Circulation 1954;**10**:481–90.*

dorsiflexed sufficiently to obtain relaxation of the wrist, such that only the lightest pressure is exerted upon the artery.

Flush

Gaertner, cited by Geddes,[23] noted that a limb blanched by occlusion flushed when the occluding pressure was released, and elaborated this finding by measuring the pressure in a finger cuff at which the flushing occurred. The principle was exploited in Blauel's apparatus.[18] Whilst the technique is attractive, it has been restricted in clinical practice to paediatric application,[24-29] and this only as a result of difficulty in obtaining satisfactory results from auscultatory methods. It has been described by Goldring[24] and the procedure in an infant requires that a cuff 5 cm in width is applied to the wrist or ankle and the limb raised to permit gross drainage of blood. A rubber bandage is applied to effect exsanguination and the cuff is inflated to some 200 mm Hg. The bandage is then removed and the cuff pressure reduced slowly. When the blanched extremity of hand or foot flushes on reperfusion, the cuff pressure is taken to reflect the systolic pressure. The appreciation of flushing is rather subjective, being affected by whether the peripheral vessels are dilated or constricted, on the haemoglobin level and on the presence or absence of local oedema. Moss *et al.*[12] provide an interesting overview.

The limb (usually an arm) is elevated for some five minutes, after which the circulation is occluded by the inflation of a cuff to a level above that of the expected systolic pressure. The cuff is then deflated slowly and the pressure in the cuff noted when the limb distal to the point of occlusion flushes.

Auscultation

Auscultation[30] is a technique based on the appreciation, via a stethoscope, of the quality of audible sound resulting from turbulence generated in a previously occluded blood vessel when the occlusion is gradually released. It is dealt with in Chapter 5.

Plethysmography

Plethysmography implies charting of changes in the volume of a tissue mass. The term dates from the time when this was one of the few methods of obtaining information about limb perfusion. The limb was enclosed in a rigid container otherwise filled with a gas or a liquid and changes in liquid volume (by displacement) or in pressure enabled inferences to be drawn about the blood supply to the limb.

More recently, the principle has been applied to determining the perfusion of a digit and, by extension, to the changes in perfusion accompanying each pulse of blood through the vessels of a finger. A beam of light, for example from a light-emitting diode (LED), is directed through the finger, to fall upon a light detector such as a photo-cell or light-detecting diode. The change in optical density due to the change in perfusion is manifest as a changing electrical signal which can be amplified and displayed; or, more simply, each signal peak may be used as a basis for counting the pulse frequency.

Devices intended to use the principle of plethysmography have been used extensively in research, but have found much less favour in clinical practice. They work by estimating or measuring the change in volume of an enclosed limb or digit, usually by displacement of gas or liquid or by change in pressure within the enclosure. With suitable care, accurate estimations may be made. However, the nature of the apparatus, its unwieldiness and the exacting conditions of measurement militate against its general use. Consequently, few commercial designs have emerged for use outside the laboratory.

Oscillometry and oscillotonometry

Oscillometry entails sensing of the pressures in an occlusive limb cuff with analogue or digital indication of the pressures corresponding to the systolic and diastolic blood pressures. The digital form is generally employed, especially in recent automated oscillometric devices.

In oscillotonometry, the changes in pressure transmitted to a sensing cuff, applied to a limb distally to an occlusive cuff as the latter is released, may be used as the basis for analogue or digital indication of the occlusion pressures corresponding to the systolic and diastolic blood pressures. When the analogue form of indication is used, a common presentation is that of a needle, moving in an arc against a background graduated scale, where the arc traversed by the needle is proportional to the change in pressure with each pulse sensed. The devices using the principle are oscillotonometers.

Both methods of monitoring are discussed in Chapter 6.

The force-balance principle

A recent technique measures the changing pressure necessary to balance the change in pressure occurring with each arterial pulsation and enables the pressures corresponding to the systolic and diastolic pressures to be derived. The principle and its application to monitoring, together with some related methods of tonometry are described in Chapter 7.

Ultrasonic pulse detection devices

The Doppler ultrasound principle has been used in the detection of the pulse in connection with sphygmomanometry (see Chapter 5) and further exploited in devices which seek to correlate changes in flow velocity with the contour of the pulse wave. The data obtained may be processed to yield systolic, diastolic, mean and other derived values.

Sensors using the principle may be secured over peripheral arteries,[31-35] usually in conjunction with a cuff. The method has found particular favour in monitoring of the blood pressure in children[36] and in neonates,[37] but may be used virtually anywhere. An unusual application is monitoring in a hyperbaric chamber[38] to which it is eminently well suited. A laser Doppler

64

technique has been described recently,[39] and Doppler measurements have been compared with those obtained by pulse oximetry.[40]

The brachial artery has been chosen as the site for the ultrasonic sensor in several commercial instruments. A single transducer both emits the ultrasound signal and detects its return. It thus behaves as a transceiver. The signal is arranged to impinge on the arterial wall and is thus susceptible to movement of the vessel wall when reflected.

The technique is highly susceptible to interference from movement artefact and other environmental factors. Moreover, the signal must be closely controlled. The interface between transducer and patient is critical to useful measurement. In particular, ultrasound is conducted very poorly through air. To this end, a liquid or semisolid interface is assured by means of liquid or gel. The quality of signals is commensurate with the care taken in application of the gel, the application of the transducer and its fixing in position.

Besides being used for the detection of blood flow and vessel wall movement in the monitoring of blood pressure, Doppler ultrasound has found new applications in non-invasive cardiovascular monitoring (see Chapter 13).

Other detectors

Other methods of detecting the pulse are used. They include:

- crystals which can sense the vibration of the vessel wall directly;
- strain gauges and microphones placed over the artery;
- finger cuffs;
- photoelectric devices.

All are position-sensitive and subject to movement artefact, although the finger cuff is placed on a phalanx of a finger and the photoelectric device is usually used on the terminal phalanx, where it is easier to secure a satisfactory position. Photoelectric sensors have commonly been used simply to detect the pulse and calculate the pulse rate (see also Chapter 12).

Special considerations

Errors and problems in blood pressure monitoring are covered in Chapter 8 and the scope and limitations of the various methods are discussed in Chapter 9, whilst ambulatory and home blood pressure monitoring are dealt with in Chapters 10 and 11, respectively.

1 Harvey W. *Exertatio Anatomica De Motu Cordis et Sanguinis in Animalibus*. Birmingham, Classics of Medicine facsimile of the 1628 edition, 1978.
2 McMullen ET. Anatomy of a physiological discovery: William Harvey and the circulation of the blood. *J Roy Soc Med* 1995; **88**, 491–8.
3 Hales S. *Statistical Essays: containing Haemostaticks*. London, Innys & Manby, 1733.
4 Booth J. A short history of blood pressure measurement. *Proc Roy Soc Med* 1977; **70**: 793–9. (Contains illustrations of Hales' experiment with the horse, Ludwig's kymograph, Marey's sphygmograph, Vierordt's sphygmograph and Von Basch's sphygmomanometer and refers to the work of Potain and of Faivre.)
5 O'Brien E, Fitzgerald D. The history of indirect blood pressure measurement. In: Birkenhager WH, Reid JL, series eds. *Handbook of hypertension*. Vol. 14. O'Brien E, O'Malley K. eds. *Blood pressure measurement*. Amsterdam: Elsevier, 1991: pp 1–54.
6 Faivre J. *Études experimentales sur les lesions organiques du coeur*. Gazette Médicale de Paris 1856: pp. 726–30.
7 Marey EJ. *Physiologie experimentale*, Vol. 2. Paris: Masson, 1876.
8 Von Basch SR. Über die Messung des Blutdrucks am Menschen mittelst des Baschschen Apparates. *Z Lin Med* 1880; **2**: 79–96.
9 Riva-Rocci S. Un sfigmomanometro nuovo. *Gaz Med Torino* 1896; **47**: 981–8; **50**: 981–6; **51**: 1000–17.
10 Hill L, Barnard H. A simple and accurate form of sphygmomanometer or arterial pressure gauge contrived for clinical use. *BMJ* 1897; **ii**: 904.
11 Von Recklinghausen H. Neue Wege der Blutdruckmessung. Fünf Abhandlungen über Blutdruck und Puls in den grossen Arterien des Menschen; Zwei-Messtellen-Vergleichsmessung. Gleichheit des systilischen, Verschiedenheit des diastolischen Drucks in den grossen Arterien. *Ztschr Klin Med* 1930; **113**: 157.
12 Moss AJ, Liebling W, Austin WO Adams FH. An evaluation of the flush method for determining blood pressures in infants. *Pediatrics* 1957; **20**: 53–62.
13 Segal HN. N.C. Korotkoff – 1874–1920 – pioneer vascular surgeon. *Amer Heart J* 1976; **91**: 816–18.
14 Korotkoff NS. On methods of studying blood pressure. *Izvestiya Imperatorskoi Voenno-Meditinskoi Akademii*, St Petersburg 1905; **11**: 365–7.
15 Segall HN. How Korotkoff, the surgeon, discovered the auscultatory method of measuring arterial pressure. *Ann Intern Med* 1975; **83**: 561–2.
16 Hutton P, Clutton-Brock TH. The non-invasive measurement of blood pressure. In: Hutton P, Prys-Roberts C, eds. *Monitoring in anaesthesia and intensive care*. London: WB Saunders Company Ltd, 1994: 106.
17 Janeway TC. *The clinical study of blood pressure*. New York: Appleton, 1904.
18 Gallavardin L. *La tension artérielle*, 2nd edn. Paris: Masson, 1920.
19 Ludwig C. Beitrage zur Kenntniss des Einflusses der Respirations bewegungen auf den Blutlauf on Aortensysteme. *Muller Arch Anat* 1847: 240–302.
20 Sykes MK, Vickers MD, Hull CJ. *Principles of measurement and monitoring in anaesthesia and intensive care*, 3rd edn. Oxford: Blackwell Scientific Publications, 1991: 69–91.
21 Bruner JRM, Krenis LJ, Kunsman JM, Sherman AP. Comparison of direct and indirect measurements of measuring arterial pressure. *Med Instrum* 1981; **15**: 11–21.
22 Van Bergen FH, Weatherhead DS, Treloar AE, Dobkin AB, Buckley JJ. Comparison of indirect and direct methods of measuring arterial pressure. *Circulation* 1954; **10**: 481–90.
23 Geddes LA. *The direct and indirect measurement of blood pressure*. Chicago: Year Book, 1970.
24 Goldring D, Wohltmann H. Flush method for blood pressure determinations in newborn infants. *J Pediatr* 1952; **40**: 285–9.
25 Cappe BE, Pallin IM. Systolic blood pressure determination in the newborn infant. *Anesthesiology* 1952; **13**: 648.
26 Sullivan MP, Kobayashi M. Evaluation of the flush technique for the determination of blood pressure in infancy. *Pediatrics* 1955; **15**: 84.
27 Reinhold J, Pym M. The determination of blood pressure by the flush method. *Arch Dis Child* 1955; **30**: 127.
28 Forfar JO, Kibel MA. Blood pressure in the newborn estimated by the flush method. *Arch Dis Child* 1956; **31**: 126.

29 Elseed AM, Shinebourne EA, Joseph MC. Assessment of techniques for measurement of blood pressure in infants and children. *Arch Dis Child* 1973; **48**: 932–6.

30 Goodman EH, Howell AA. Clinical studies in the auscultatory method of determining blood pressure. *Univ Penn Med Bull* 1911; **23**: 469–75.

31 Greenfield ADM, Whitney RJ, Mowbray JF. Methods for the investigation of peripheral blood flow. *Br Med Bull* 1963; **19**: 101–9.

32 Kirby RR, Kemmerer WT, Morgan JL. Transcutaneous Doppler measurement of blood pressure. *Anesthesiology* 1969; **31**: 86–9.

33 Stegall HF, Kardon MB, Kemmerer WT. Direct measurement of arterial blood pressure by Doppler ultrasonic sphygmomanometry. *J Appl Physiol* 1968; **25**: 793–8.

34 Kazamias TM, Gander MP, Franklin DL, Ross J. Blood pressure measurement with the Doppler ultrasonic flowmeter. *J Appl Physiol* 1971; **30**: 585–8.

35 Waltemath CL, Preuss DD. Determination of blood pressure in low flow states by the Doppler technique. *Anesthesiology* 1971; **34**: 77–9.

36 Zahed B, Sadove MS, Hatano S, Wu HH. Comparison of automated Doppler ultrasound and Korotkoff measurements of blood pressure of children. *Anesth Analg* 1971; **50**: 699–704.

37 Emery EF, Greenough A. Non-invasive blood pressure monitoring in preterm infants receiving intensive care. *Eur J Pediatr* 1992; **151**: 136–9.

38 Weaver LK, Howe S. Noninvasive Doppler blood pressure monitoring in the monoplace hyperbaric chamber. *J Clin Monit* 1991; **7**: 304–8.

39 Beinder E, Hoffmann U, Franzeck UK, Huch A, Huch R, Bollinger A. Laser Doppler technique for the measurement of digital and segmental systolic blood pressure. *Vasa* 1992; **21**: 15–21.

40 Wallace CT, Baker JD, Alpert CC, Tankersley SJ, Conroy JM, Kerns RE. Comparison of blood pressure measurements by Doppler and by pulse oximetry techniques. *Anesth Analg* 1987; **66**: 1018–19.

5 Sphygmomanometry

The definition by Korotkoff of a series of sounds during auscultation of the pulse denoting phases of the cuff deflation pressure was a major advance in the indirect measurement of blood pressure. Controversy still surrounds the interpretation of the significance of the sounds and it is instructive, first of all, to recapitulate the description given by Korotkoff and elaborated by Goodman and Howell.[1] They described five sounds, termed "phases", as shown in the box below.

Auscultation

The basis of the sounds thus described is attributed to vibrations set up in the wall of the artery as the contained blood undergoes differing degrees of turbulence in the face of partial occlusion or deformation of the vessel.

These vibrations are most commonly detected as sound by auscultation through a stethoscope applied to the brachial artery at the elbow, but other methods of detection are used, especially when the process is automated (q.v.). Other sites, such as over the radial popliteal and posterior tibial arteries, may be used but are generally less convenient than the brachial artery. It may be argued that sound production may be delayed until blood flow is properly established and that some of the sound may be absorbed by the tissues intervening between artery and stethoscope, but these considerations may be neglected for practical purposes.

There is general agreement about the point at which the sound corresponding to the systolic pressure may be heard. Its appearance is generally clear cut and cannot be confused with any other sound generated at a pressure close to the systolic.

Auscultation – Korotkoff's sounds

- Phase I   Sudden appearance of tapping sounds
- Phase II Sounds become quieter (pulse palpable at wrist)
- Phase III Sounds become louder and tapping
- Phase IV Muffling (high frequency components disappear)
- Phase V   Sounds are absent

It should be noted that the shape of the envelope containing the acoustic waveform denotes a rapid onset and a sharp rise to the maximum amplitude. Much of the frequency range of the Korotkoff sounds falls outside that of human hearing. In subjects who are hypotensive or atherosclerotic they may in any case be difficult to hear.

The tapping nature of the sounds when they first appear at the pressure corresponding to systole are thought to be due to the high-frequency components of the vibration in a taut vessel wall. Similarly, those sounds with a similar character near the diastolic point contain a predominance of high frequencies. In between, the vessel wall pressure gradient across the arterial wall is less and lower frequencies predominate. Once the diastolic pressure has been passed, the lower frequencies still predominate, though not so noticeably.

Mention should be made here of the auscultatory gap, first described by Cook and Taussig in 1917.[2] It sometimes happens that the characteristic sounds are absent over a range of values between the systolic and diastolic pressures. The consequence of this is that if the cuff is inflated to a pressure within this range and the auscultatory method then used for detection of the systolic point, this will be incorrectly identified at the lower extremity of the auscultatory gap (q.v.) in the sounds.

The diastolic pressure is much less easy to establish. Opinions have long been divided and the merits of the fading of the fifth sound versus its total disappearance have occupied many authorities.[3-9] The matter was addressed by the American Heart Association,[10] who recommended at that time that Phase IV, the end-point then also popular in the UK, be used.

Arguments in favour Phase IV as the end-point include:

- theoretical reasons for believing that the change from a full sound to a muffled sound should correspond to the diastolic pressure;
- the uncertainty associated with identifying the point at which sounds may be said to have faded when Phase V is used (it is thought to be largely subjective);
- the fact, already mentioned, that some patients' sounds do not disappear until a very low pressure is attained, certainly well below that at which muffling occurs (for example, in pregnancy and other high cardiac output states and in the elderly).[11]

Against Phase IV are:

- in comparative studies, the directly measured diastolic pressure has more closely corresponded to Phase V;
- Phase V seems more readily identified by most studies, where observations correlate well.[10,12]

More recently, however, extensive studies have made the case for Phase V in adults and Phase IV in children, the position now adopted by the

American Heart Association.[13] O'Brien and his colleagues, however, confirm the recommendations of the World Health Organisation in 1962 that both Phase IV and Phase V pressures be recorded for hypertension research.[12]

Validity of sphygmomanometry

A number of comparisons have been made between sphygmomanometric readings and data obtained from direct arterial blood pressure measurements.[11,14–20] In practice, the rate of deflation of the cuff and interference from variations in the heart rate and the respiratory pattern, render such comparisons of limited value in relation to individual blood pressure estimations.

Apparatus

The apparatus consists of an inflatable cuff provided with an inflating bulb and manually operated valve for the occlusion of the vessel in the arm or leg and a manometer, either a mercury manometer or an aneroid gauge.

The mercury manometer consists of a glass column containing mercury in continuity with a mercury reservoir that is in communication with the inflatable cuff. The column is calibrated in mm Hg. Since mercury is approximately 13 times as heavy as water, the problems of a water column which would need to be 13 times higher are avoided. (Note: 1 mm Hg = 0.133 kPa (beware literal translations) and 1 cm water or isotonic saline = 0.74 mm Hg.)

The mercury column has long been regarded as a standard against which other manometers could be judged in sphygmomanometry. However, its use in *routine* sphygmomanometry has come under scrutiny by Stewart and Padfield[21] who, in an extensive review of the subject and, whilst accepting that for the time being alternatives are often unreliable in practice, conclude that "new methods of BP measurements being developed may improve the diagnostic accuracy of such devices further ... and may yet replace the mercury sphygmomanometer". The context is largely that of home and ambulatory blood pressure monitoring, but the implication is clear nevertheless. The general progress already made six years before their statement was reviewed by Sanford and coworkers.[22] Stewart and Padfield have meanwhile been looking towards what the future may hold.[23]

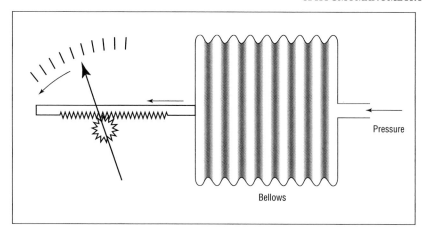

Figure 5.1 A low pressure aneroid gauge.[D]

The aneroid manometer (Figure 5.1) was devised to measure pressure without the necessity for a column of liquid. It originally took the form of a metal chamber with extensive end surfaces such that pressure exerted from within the chamber caused the ends to bow. One end-plate was fixed and the other was connected via a linkage to an indicating pointer. The chamber now more commonly takes the form of a metal bellows into which the pressure from the cuff is admitted. Here again, one end of the bellows is fixed and the other end is linked to a pointer. The pointer moves against a dial calibrated in mm Hg.

The accuracy of aneroid gauges has often been called into question,[24,25] but it has to be said that they suffer badly from lack of regular maintenance and calibration.[26] Some of the mechanical shortcomings of mercury sphygmomanometers, such as mercury leaks, inflating valve defects and leaking air tubing, are also traceable to misuse and poor or absent maintenance.[27]

Method

Assuming that the brachial artery has been chosen as the site of measurement, a baseline measurement should be made. The subject should be made comfortable and the arm positioned in such a way that the point of auscultation is on a level with the heart. Measurements should be made in both arms, since the results may differ, perhaps indicating a pathological abnormality,[28] and the question will arise as to which reading constitutes a valid base line estimation.

The sphygmomanometer used should be in good condition and well maintained. It should be placed in a position where the observer can view

KOROTKOFF SOUNDS

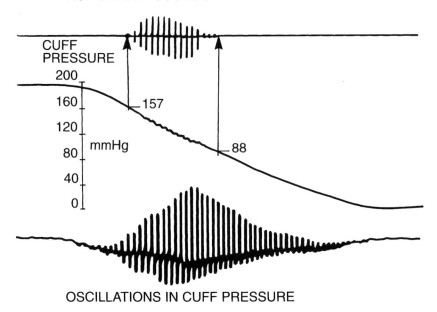

OSCILLATIONS IN CUFF PRESSURE

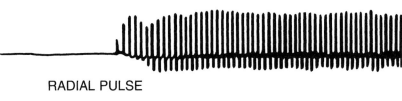

RADIAL PULSE

5 SEC.

Figure 5.2 The effect of cuff fit on blood pressure reading. (1) When a blood pressure cuff of proper width is snugly applied, the tissue pressure around deep arteries under the cuff equals the cuff pressure; (2) A cuff that is too narrow in relation to the diameter of the limb does not transmit its pressure to the centre of the limb, so that cuff pressure must exceed arterial pressure to produce occlusion of the artery and falsely high systolic and diastolic pressures may be read. A loose cuff also results in artefactual elevation of the blood pressure. Note: A cuff that is too wide, although bulky, is unlikely to distort the readings.[B,F]

it and apply a stethoscope without undue strain or discomfort. It is important that the procedure be unhurried.

The cuff which is selected must be appropriate to the arm to which it is to be applied,[29-35] i.e. it should have the dimensions specified for different circumferences of limb (see box overleaf and Figure 5.2). So long as the *width* of the cuff is at least 12 cm and the *length* at least 40 cm, errors due to imperfect width are likely to be minor.[36] Ideally, it should have a mark identifying that part of the cuff which should lie immediately over the

72

Important factors in the auscultatory method of blood pressure measurement

- Sphygmomanometer should be in good condition and well maintained.
- Cuff should be the correct size (i.e. bladder length should be 80% and its width 40%, respectively, of arm circumference).
- Use the bell of the stethoscope rather than the diaphragm.
- Get the subject comfortable and place the sphygmomanometer where you can see the scale and take the reading comfortably.
- Be unhurried – confirm the expected systolic pressure level by palpation and deflate the cuff *slowly* (no faster than 3 mm Hg per second).
- For a baseline reading, remember to measure the blood pressure in both arms.

brachial artery. It should be applied closely, although not tightly.[37] The cuff need not encircle the arm. However, wrap-around cuffs lend themselves to being placed and secured correctly. Cuffs which are too small or too loose are prone to giving falsely high readings; and, conversely, those which are too large or are applied too tightly may yield readings which are too low.[38] Obese patients are particularly susceptible to erroneous readings due to the application of inappropriate cuffs,[39-41] and measurements in the elderly require careful consideration of cuff size and security,[42] especially if what is known as "pseudohypertension" is not to be diagnosed inadvertently.[43-46] The extent to which small and large cuffs are in agreement has been re-examined recently.[47]

Whether or not the cuff needs to encircle the arm is disputed,[34,39,48] although the point has been made that perhaps cuff encirclement of the arm matters less than placing the cuff directly over the artery.[29] Further influences are the rate at which the cuff is inflated and deflated,[49-51] and the particular characteristics of the stethoscope employed in auscultation.[52] Whatever the arguments about these matters, it has been stated that practical difficulties would be few if the current guidelines were followed properly.[53]

Some cuffs have markings to indicate exactly where they should be placed in relation to the artery.

The pulse at the wrist should be palpated to determine whether or not the rhythm is regular, as abnormalities of rhythm may indicate variations in cardiac output and, hence, in the blood pressure, that might occur during the course of a single blood pressure estimation. The brachial pulse should next be located and the bell of the stethoscope placed over it. The bell is preferred to the diaphragm because the Korotkoff sounds occupy a relatively low frequency range in relation to that of human hearing and the bell is better suited to these low frequencies, whilst sounds of higher frequency from the movement of a diaphragm on the skin are eliminated.

For best results, the bell of the stethoscope must be placed directly over the artery. To secure this position and to maintain it for the duration of the blood pressure measurement, it is necessary to support the subject's arm satisfactorily. As has been noted, although diaphragm stethoscopes or attachments are often seen in practice, they cannot generally be recommended for auscultation of the Korotkoff sounds. An exception may be made under emergency conditions and when access is difficult, e.g. when it is convenient to attach a stethoscope to the auscultation site during monitoring of a patient covered by sterile towels as, for example, during local anaesthesia. However, the use of an automated remote device is recommended in the latter instance.

Amplified stethoscopes are available which aid the appreciation and interpretation of the heart and chest sounds. It is doubtful whether the amplification confers significant benefit in arterial auscultation and the caveat concerning diaphragms also holds.

The valve adjacent to the inflating bulb is fully closed and the cuff is inflated quickly to some 30 mm Hg above the expected systolic pressure (a rough guide being some 30 mm Hg above that at which the pressure in the cuff occludes the radial pulse, which becomes impalpable). When the range of the readings is unknown, it is usual to inflate the cuff to between 250 and 300 mm Hg and then deflate the cuff relatively quickly whilst palpating the artery and noting the pressure at which pulsations reappear. Measurements are then carried out by inflating to some 30 mm Hg above this pressure. The cuff is then deflated slowly by opening the valve only slightly, so that the pressure indicated by the column declines by no more than 3 mm Hg per second (ideally, about 2 mm Hg per second).

The reason for limiting the rate of fall of the cuff pressure is that, at a normal heart rate of around 70 beats per minute, a more rapid fall risks misinterpretation of the first genuine pulse, as opposed to that of the pulse producing the first sound at a steady cuff pressure. Thus, during a more rapid rate of fall, the systolic pressure is likely to be interpreted at a falsely low level. It follows that the likelihood of this kind of error is reduced when the heart rate is lower than normal and increased when it is higher.

The first sound to be heard, as already noted, is the first "tapping" Korotkoff sound (Figure 5.3), the advent of which is usually clear and distinct (Korotkoff Phase I). The pressure at this point is taken to denote the systolic arterial pressure. As the cuff is deflated further, the sound becomes more full at first, but later declines in amplitude and, subsequently, changes in character. The pulse becomes palpable at the wrist at a pressure close to the systolic pressure (Phase II). As the cuff pressure is further released, the sounds become tapping in character once again (Phase III). The point at which either the sounds become muffled (Phase IV) or disappear (Phase V) is variously interpreted as the diastolic arterial blood

74

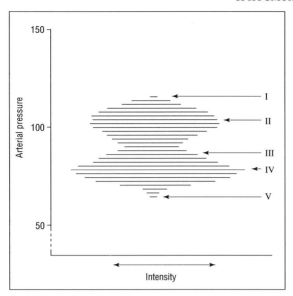

Figure 5.3 Diagrammatic representation of the Korotkoff sounds, showing intensity in relation to each of the five sounds.[C]

pressure. The pressures in Phases IV and V are usually separated by some 5–10 mm Hg. However, in some subjects, the sounds may not disappear until the pressures are very low indeed, even approaching zero. Considerable debate has taken place concerning the correct interpretation of the Korotkoff sounds when the diastolic point is approached. Several factors emerge, however:

- the nature and rate of the change in the character of the sound is different in different subjects;
- the change of character may be forestalled by disappearance of the sound altogether;
- authorities have disagreed on whether "muffling" or disappearance of the sounds should be regarded as the definitive correlative of the diastolic point.

In this last regard, some authorities have referred to a three-component measurement based upon the systolic sound, the muffled diastolic sound and the disappearance of the sounds, as opposed to the two-component approach recognising simply the systolic sound and the diastolic sound. Fortunately, the subject has been reviewed and recommendations made in respect of conditions in the UK and the USA.[54–56]

75

Problems encountered during measurement

Obesity

Use of an unsuitably small cuff bladder results in over-reading, thus yielding a falsely high estimation. Even when an appropriate cuff is applied in obese subjects, the interposition of excessive tissue renders the reading more dubious and may present problems when considered to be on the margin of hypertension.[39]

"Mutton" arms

This is a term sometimes used to describe short and fat cone-shaped arms, to which it may be difficult to apply a cuff satisfactorily. An alternative is to place the cuff on the forearm and attempt auscultation over the radial artery at the wrist.

Auscultatory gap

The auscultatory gap (Figure 5.4) is the term used to describe a zone in the pressure range between the systolic and diastolic pressures in some individuals in which no sounds can be heard.[57] The condition is particularly prevalent in hypertensive subjects who, although they are indeed hypertensive, may have diastolic pressures attributed to them which are falsely high, if based on the disappearance of the sounds constituting the "gap". Whenever the sounds disappear altogether and especially when this happens in known hypertensives and/or at relatively high pressures, it is important to allow the pressure to decline further and to listen with the stethoscope for the possible reappearance of the sounds. Similarly, the possibility of recording a falsely low systolic pressure, by first starting to release the cuff pressure within the auscultatory gap, may be avoided by ensuring that the cuff is inflated to some 30 mm Hg above the point at which the radial pulse is lost to palpation. It is therefore essential that the cuff be inflated to a pressure such that the pulse is occluded (and, hence, impalpable) *before* auscultation is undertaken, so as to avoid the problem.

Respiratory variation

The volume of the pulse may be seen to be greater during inspiration than during expiration in normal subjects, although the range of this variation is usually less than 10 mm Hg.

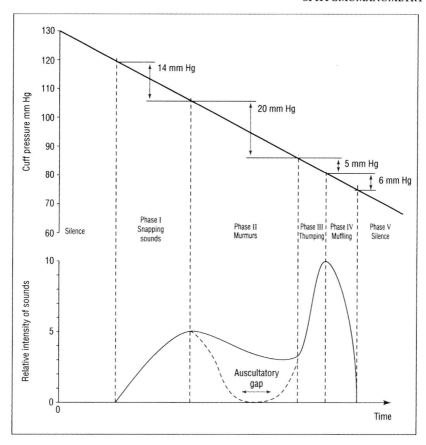

Figure 5.4 Relative intensity of the Korotkoff sounds at different cuff pressures. Note the auscultatory gap.[A]

Pulsus alternans is the term used to describe a pulse pattern in which every second beat is of greater amplitude than its predecessor.

Pulsus paradoxus refers to the condition in which the blood pressure varies during breathing but, in this instance, the systolic level is higher during expiration than during inspiration. The difference between the normal condition and pulsus paradoxus is therefore determined by asking the patient to breathe normally and noting whether the systolic sound is first evident, during *very slow* deflation of the cuff, in inspiration or expiration. Continuing to deflate the cuff and taking readings will establish the point at which the sounds can be heard in both phases of breathing and the pressure noted. The difference between this pressure and the pressure at which the sounds first appeared in either phase is known as the systolic gradient.

77

Circumstances in which auscultatory readings may be misleading

Over-reading

- Arm too low in relation to the heart (common practice)
- Cuff too small or too tight
- Cuff imperfectly placed, e.g. not properly placed over the artery
- Subject obese and/or inappropriate cuff too small – if subject grossly obese, try a thigh cuff on the upper arm
- Awkwardly shaped arm – try forearm or leg

Under-reading

- Cuff too large
- Arm too high (though improbable)
- Cuff deflation too fast (remember – not more than 3 mm Hg/sec)
- Starting measurements in auscultatory gap – make sure cuff is inflated to a pressure above that at which the corresponding pulse becomes impalpable

A variant, *reversed pulsus paradoxus*, in which the systolic pressure rises during inspiration, has been described in patients subjected to automatic ventilation when hypovolaemic.

Pulsus bisferiens is an uncommon condition in which each arterial pulse has two peaks. The first is due to cardiac ejection in early systole and the second to a surge of flow in late systole. It is found in patients with mixed aortic stenosis and regurgitation, and the peaks may be equal in amplitude or the first greater than the second.

Some practical considerations

Although this method is often accorded the status of "routine" and hence prone to be delegated on the basis of seeing it done and then going away and doing it, the use of sphygmomanometry, in circumstances where accuracy is required, demands a more rigorous approach. The importance of accurate measurements, for example, in the assessment and follow-up monitoring of hypertensive patients and in the preoperative assessment of patients who are to undergo general anaesthesia cannot be overemphasised.

The sitting or lying patient

The recumbent patient at rest in bed or on an examination couch may present few problems, in that the arm is at or about the level of the heart and may well be resting on the bed or couch and, thus, be in a stable position. More often, the subject is not lying down. Try to avoid estimations in subjects who are standing; they should be seated comfortably with access to a surface on which the arm can be conveniently supported. The temptation to ask the patient to hold the arm out in space or to support it under the operator's own arm must be resisted. Under these conditions, the occlusive cuff should be very close to the level of the heart. Differences in the actual position achieved may be expected to have only a very minor effect on the validity of the reading obtained, since each 1·3 cm above or below the optimum level represents a potential error of just 1 mm Hg.

Movement artefacts

Although gross movements are easily appreciated, progressive movements due to pressure of the stethoscope on an unsupported or poorly supported arm are less obvious. The nature of the rim of the bell-ended stethoscope renders it less prone to movement and slipping than the diaphragm which, when moved, produces distracting crackles and is in any case less satisfactory for arterial auscultation than the bell.

Physical constraints

Physical deformities, injuries and obesity may make the application of cuffs difficult or impossible at certain sites. When undue difficulty is encountered or when there is reason to question the probable validity of readings on these grounds, another site should be selected. Cuffs are available for use on the thigh and the differences between the values obtained at this site and those obtained from the arm are small.

1 Goodman EH, Howell AA. Further clinical studies in the auscultatory method of determining blood pressure. *Amer J Med Sci* 1911; **142**: 344.
2 Cook JE, Taussig AE. Auscultatory blood pressure determination, a source of possible error. *JAMA* 1917; **68**: 1088.
3 London SB, London RE. Critique of indirect diastolic end-point. *Arch Intern Med* 1967; **119**: 39–49.
4 King GE. Recommendations for sphygmomanometry. A dissenting opinion. *Am Heart J* 1969; **77**: 147–8.
5 Short D. The diastolic dilemma. *BMJ* 1975; **ii**: 685–6.
6 Folsom AR, Prineas RJ, Jacobs DR, Leupker RV, Gillum RF. Measured differences between fourth and fifth phase diastolic blood pressures in 4885 adults: implications for blood pressure surveys. *Int J Epidemiol* 1984; **13**: 436–41.
7 Manek S, Rutherford J, Jackson SHD, Turner P. Persistence of divergent views of hospital staff in detecting and managing hypertension. *BMJ* 1984; **289**: 1433–4.
8 Hense H-W, Stieber J, Chambless L. Factors associated with measured differences between fourth and fifth phase diastolic blood pressure. *Int J Epidemiol* 1986; **15**: 513–18.

9 Lichtenstein MJ, Rose G, Shipley M. Distribution and determination of the difference between diastolic phase 4 and phase 5 blood pressure. *J Hypertens* 1986; **4**: 361–3.

10 Kirkendall WM, Burton AC, Epstein FH, Freis ED. *Recommendations for human blood pressure determination by sphygmomanometers*. Subcommittee of the AHA Postgraduate Education Committee, American Heart Association. *Circulation* 1967; **36**: 980–8.

11 Van Bergen FH, Weatherhead DS, Treloar AE, Dobkin AB, Buckley JJ. Comparison of indirect and direct methods of measuring arterial pressure. *Circulation* 1954; **10**: 481–90.

12 O'Brien ET, Beevers DG, Marshall HJ. *ABC of Hypertension*, 3rd edn. London: BMJ Publishing Group, 1995: p. 25.

13 Kirkendall WM, Feinlieb M, Freis, ED, Mark AL. *Recommendations for human blood pressure determination by sphygmomanometers*. Subcommittee of the AHA Postgraduate Education Committee, American Heart Association. *Circulation* 1980; **62**: 1146A–55A.

14 Pereira E, Prys-Roberts C, Dagnino J, Anger C, Cooper GM, Hutton P. Auscultatory measurement of arterial pressure during anaesthesia: a reassessment of Korotkoff sounds. *Eur J Anaesth* 1985; **2**: 11–20.

15 Hunyor SN, Flynn JM, Cochineas C. Comparison of various sphygmomanometers with intra-arterial blood pressure readings. *BMJ* 1978; **iii**: 159–62.

16 Berliner K, Fujiy H, Ho Lee D. Yildiz M, Garnier B. The accuracy of blood pressure determinations: a comparison of direct and indirect measurements. *Cardiologica* 1960; **37**: 118–28.

17 Holland WW, Humerfelt S. Measurements of blood pressure: comparison of intra-arterial and cuff values. *BMJ* 1964; **ii**: 1241–3.

18 Henschel A, de la Vega F., Taylor HL. Simultaneous direct and indirect blood pressure measurements in man at rest and work. *J Appl Physiol* 1954; **6**: 506–8.

19 Vardan S, Mookherjee S, Warner R, Smulyan H. Systolic hypertension. Direct and indirect measurements. *Arch Intern Med* 1983; **143**: 935–8.

20 O'Callaghan WG, Fitzgerald DJ, O'Malley K, O'Brien E. Accuracy of indirect blood pressure measurement in the elderly. *BMJ* 1983; **286**: 1545–6.

21 Stewart MJ, Padfield PL. Blood pressure measurement: an epitaph for the mercury sphygmomanometer. *Clin Sci* 1992; **83**: 1–12.

22 Sanford TJ, Jones BR, Smith NT. Noninvasive blood pressure measurement. *Anesthesiol Clin N Am* 1986; **6**: 671.

23 Stewart MJ, Padfield PL. Measurement of blood pressure in the technological age. *Br Med Bull* 1994; **50**: 420–42.

24 Bowman C. Blood pressure errors with aneroid sphygmomanometers. *Lancet* 1981; **i**: 1005.

25 Patee JR, Rose D. Aneroid sphygmomanometers. Are they accurate monitors of blood pressure? *Anesthesiol Rev* 1981; **8**: 42–4.

26 Perlman LV, Chiang BN, Keller J, Blackburn H. Accuracy of sphygmomanometers in hospital practice. *Arch Int Med* 1970; 1000–3.

27 Conceico S, Ward MK, Kerr DNS. Defects in sphygmomanometers: an important source of error in blood pressure recording. *BMJ* 1976; **i**: 886–8.

28 Gould BA, Hornung RS, Kieso HA, Altman DG, Raftery EB. Is the blood pressure the same in both arms? *Clin Cardiol* 1985; **8**: 423–6.

29 Burch GE, Shewey L. Sphygmomanometric cuff size and blood pressure recordings. *JAMA* 1973; **225**: 1215–18.

30 Croft PR, Cruikshank JK. Blood pressure measurement in adults: large cuffs for all? *N Engl Med J* 1990; **44**: 170–3.

31 Geddes LA, Whistler S. The error in indirect blood pressure measurement with the incorrect cuff size. *Amer Heart J* 1978; **96**: 4–8.

32 Karvonen MJ, Telivuo LJ, Jarvinen EJK. Sphygmomanometer cuff size and accuracy of indirect blood pressure determination. *Amer J Cardiol* 1964; **13**: 688–93.

33 Russell AE, Wing LMH, Smith SA *et al*. Optimal size of cuff bladder for indirect measurement of arterial pressure in adults. *J Hypertension* 1989; 7: 607–14.

34 Simpson JA, Jamieson G, Dickhaus DW, Grover RF. Effect of size of cuff bladder on accuracy of measurement of indirect blood pressure. *Amer Heart J* 1965; **70**: 208–15.

35 Whincup PH, Cook DG, Shaper AG. Blood pressure measurement in children: the importance of cuff size. *J Hypertens* 1989; 7: 845–50.

36 O'Brien ET, Beevers DG, Marshall HJ. *ABC of Hypertension*, 3rd edn. London: BMJ Publishing Group, 1995: p. 12.

37 Banner TE, Gravenstein JS. How tightly to wrap a blood pressure cuff. *Anesthesiology* 1990; **71**: A352.

38 Stolt M, Sjonell G, Astrom H, Hansson L. The reliability of auscultatory measurement of arterial blood pressure. A comparison of the standard and a new methodology. *Amer J Hypertens* 1990; **3**: 697–703.

39 King GE. Errors in clinical measurement of blood pressure in obesity. *Clin Sci* 1967; **32**: 223–37.

40 Linfors EW, Feussner JR, Blessing CL, Starmer CF, Neelon FA, McKee PA. Spurious hypertension in the obese patient. Effect of sphygmomanometer cuff size on prevalence of hypertension. *Arch Int Med* 1984; **144**: 1482–5.

41 Maxwell MH, Waks AU, Schroth PC, Karam M, Dornfeld LP. Error in blood pressure measurement due to incorrect cuff size in obese patients. *Lancet* 1982; **ii**: 33–6.

42 O'Callaghan, WG, Fitzgerald DJ, O'Malley K, O'Brien E. Accuracy of indirect blood pressure measurement in the elderly. *BMJ* 1983; **286**: 1545–6.

43 Taguchi JT, Suwangool P. "Pipe-stem" brachial arteries. A cause of pseudohypertension. *JAMA* 1974; **228**: 733.

44 Wallace CT, Carpenter FA, Evins SC, Mahaffey JE. Acute pseudohypertensive crisis. *Anesthesiology* 1975; **43**: 588–9.

45 Spence JD, Sibbald WJ, Cape RD. Pseudohypertension in the elderly. *Clin Sci Mol Med* 1978; **55**: 399–402S.

46 Messerli FH, Ventura HO, Amodeo C. Osler's maneuver and pseudohypertension. *N Engl J Med* 1985; **312**: 1548–51.

47 Iyriboz Y, Hearon CM, Edwards K. Agreement between large and small cuffs in sphygmomanometry: a quantitative assessment. *J Clin Monit* 1994; **10**: 127–33.

48 Steinfeld L, Alexander H, Cohen ML. Updating sphygmomanometry. *Amer J Cardiol* 1974; **33**: 107–10.

49 King GE. Influence of rate of cuff inflation and deflation on observed blood pressure by sphygmomanometry. *Amer Heart J* 1963; **65**: 303–6.

50 Fries ED, Sappington RF. Dynamic reactions produced by deflating a blood pressure cuff. *Circulation* 1968; **38**: 1085–96.

51 Yong PG, Geddes LA. The effect of cuff pressure deflation rate on accuracy in indirect measurement of blood pressure with the auscultatory method. *J Clin Monit* 1987; **3**: 155–9.

52 Whitcher CE. Stethoscope performance in transduction of human Korotkoff blood pressure sounds. *Anesthesiology* 1968; **29**: 215–16.

53 Campbell NR, McKay DW, Chockalingam A, Fodor JG. Errors in assessment of blood pressure: sphygmomanometers and blood pressure cuffs. *Can J Public Health* 1994; **85** (Suppl. 2): S22–5.

54 Petrie JC, O'Brien ET, Littler WA, de Swiet M. Recommendations on blood pressure measurement. *BMJ* 1986; **293**: 611–15.

55 Frohlich ED, Grim C. Labarthe DR, Maxwell MH, Perloff D, Weidman WH. Recommendations for human blood pressure determination by sphygmomanometers. *Hypertension* 1988; **11**: 209–22A.

56 Perloff D, Grim C, Flak J *et al.* Human blood pressure determination by sphygmomanometry: American Heart Association Medical/Scientific Statement: special report. *Circulation* 1993: **88**: 2460–70.

57 Ragan C, Bordley J. The accuracy of clinical measurements of arterial blood pressure, with a note on the auscultatory gap. *Bull Johns Hopkins Hosp* 1941; **69**: 504.

Further reading

Geddes LA. *The direct and indirect measurement of blood pressure.* Chicago: Year Book, 1970.

6 Oscillometry and oscillotonometry

Von Recklinghausen's work on indirect measurement of the blood pressure led him to define two approaches to sensing flow by means of cuffs.[1] In the first, *oscillometry*, a single cuff was used in which changes in pressure were sensed and these same changing pressures were the basis of the estimation. In the second, *oscillotonometry*, two separate cuffs were used. One, placed proximally on the arm, occluded arterial flow and subsequently permitted flow against decreasing restriction, whilst the other, placed more distally on the arm, sensed pressure changes downstream of the occlusion site. It was found that, in both systems, the pressures used for the estimation followed a distinctive pattern. First, as the pressure in a fully occlusive cuff approached and reached the systolic pressure, the very small deflection on an aneroid manometer, from tissue distortion by the arterial pulsation just proximal to the cuff, gave way to a definitive larger scale deflection. As the occluding pressure was gently released, so the deflection grew larger, but subsequently declined and virtually disappeared at the diastolic point. In the oscillotonometric method, two separate aneroid manometers measured the pressures in the proximal occluding cuff and the distal sensing cuff.

This arrangement gave place to a single aneroid manometer which sensed the pressure in the proximal cuff during occlusion and was then switched by the movement of a lever to sense the pressure in the distal cuff. The method was later refined so that the lower cuff overlapped the upper cuff. An overlap of about one third the distance across the upper cuff was found to be most satisfactory.

In recent times, both approaches have come to occupy an important place in monitoring. Oscillotonometry, in particular, has found favour with anaesthetists, whilst oscillometry has been the basis of a variety of automated monitoring and surveillance devices. The comparability of this kind of indirect approach with direct intra-arterial pressure monitoring has been investigated.

Oscillometry

The oscillometer exploits the fact that, when a sphygmomanometer cuff is deflated from a pressure above the systolic pressure of the subject, the

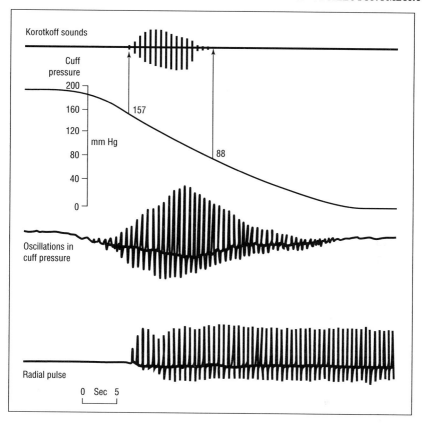

Figure 6.1 Auscultatory, oscillometric and palpatory blood pressures compared. It is impossible to determine the diastolic level from the palpatory record,[B] *and Geddes LA,* The direct and indirect measurement of blood pressure, *St Louis: Mosby – Year Book 1970.*

pulsation of the vessel, when it is no longer totally occluded, is transmitted to the occlusive cuff, thereby superimposing a pressure change (in the form of an oscillation of pressure) on the prevailing partial occlusion cuff pressure.[2,3] Although this can be discerned in feeble oscillation of the column of mercury in a mercury sphygmomanometer and in the oscillating movement of the needle of an aneroid pressure gauge, it has an amplitude insufficient to permit visual appreciation of the characteristics it represents at different points during deflation of the occluding cuff.[4] However, sensitive yet robust miniature pressure transducers made it possible to follow these oscillating pressure changes, amplify them electronically, and display them in a satisfactory manner[5,6] (Figure 6.1). Some of the transducers have been experimental only.[7–10]

Nevertheless, the principle is well documented[11–14] and is now the basis of many commercial instruments. Many blood pressure measuring

83

instruments constitute modules in assemblies of monitoring devices and, hence, need to be remote from the site of measurement and to some extent, from the hand of the operator. Because there is no necessity for operator interference, other than to inflate the occlusion system in manual instruments, these instruments have fulfilled a long-felt need.

Moreover, the nature of the technique lends itself to being harnessed to continuous deflation, without the pauses occasioned by having to hold a pressure level, whilst each observation is made as part of the set required to establish the systolic and diastolic points. The continuity of the analysis in microprocessor-based systems, now commonplace, enables artefact detection to be included in the control algorithms. The result is more rapid and, at the same time, more trouble-free monitoring.

Reasons for abandonment and rediscovery

Although oscillometry is the simpler of the two techniques, visual appreciation of the deflection produced directly from the occlusive cuff was insufficiently discriminating to permit accurate observations to be carried out. Thus, it was not popular initially. More recently, detectors have become available which are sufficiently sensitive to pressure changes and whose signals can be suitably amplified. It is this feature which has resulted in the adoption of the technique for continuous monitoring and monitoring in difficult situations. The cuffs can be rugged and can be produced inexpensively.

Oscillotonometry

The oscillotonometer is shown in Figure 6.2. The essential feature here is that a second cuff performs the sensing function, as originally described by Von Recklinghausen in 1931[15] (Figure 6.3). As in his original instrument, current adult models have an occluding cuff some 5 cm wide, whereas the sensing cuff has a width of 10 cm and overlaps the occluding cuff by approximately 2 cm. The sensing cuff is usually arranged to overlap the occluding cuff over about one-third of its width.[16] The cuffs are isolated from each other by a spring-loaded lever-operated rotary valve. In the normal position, the inflating bulb, the occluding cuff, and the sensing cuff are all in communication with the interior of the instrument which is sealed from the atmosphere. Inside the housing is an aneroid pressure-sensing chamber linked to a pointer on a dial on the face of the instrument, so that the pressure in the interior of the instrument can be indicated on the imprinted scale. This aneroid communicates with the atmosphere, so that it has a reference to atmospheric pressure. In the depressed position, in

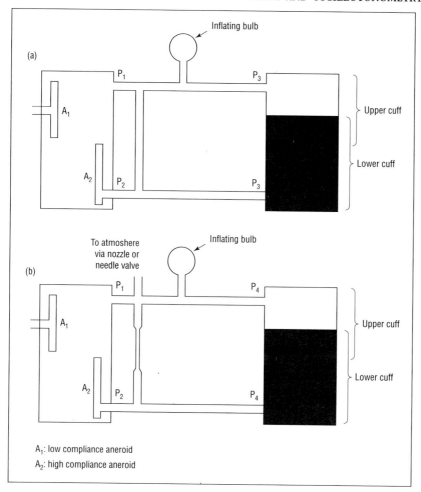

Figure 6.2 Diagrammatic representation of the principle of the oscillotonometer. (a) Represents the conditions during inflation and when cuff pressure measurement is being made; (b) Represents the conditions during deflation.[A,C] *Cited as* Br J Anaesth *1982;54:581–91.*

which it is held by finger pressure against the spring loading, the valve isolates the inflating bulb and the interior of the instrument, and permits communication between the sensing cuff and a second aneroid sensor, also situated within the instrument housing. This latter communication is large enough to allow constant near-equilibrium between the sensing cuff and its associated aneroid chamber. A linkage involving a fulcrum plate enables the second aneroid to impart oscillations due to pressure changes within it to be relayed to and superimposed upon the mechanical pressure indication derived directly from the first aneroid (Figure 6.4). The rotary valve itself has an air-bleed valve mounted upon it and operated by a knurled knob

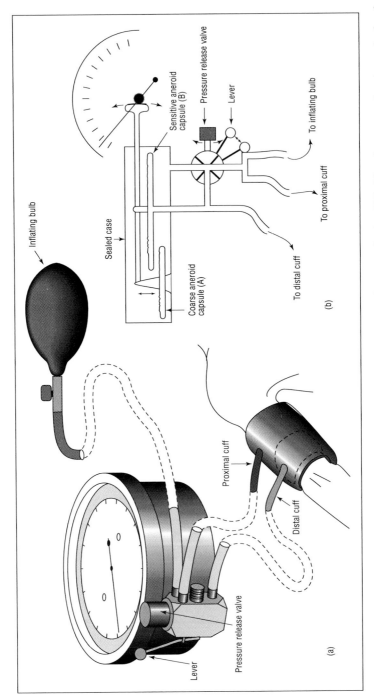

Figure 6.3 The Von Recklinghausen oscillotonometer. (a) Shows the instrument with integral pressure releasing ("bleed") valve, connected to the proximal and distal patient cuffs and to the manual inflating bulb. (b) Shows a diagrammatic section of the chamber containing the two aneroid capsules (one coarse and the other sensitive) and the manner in which communication between the inflating bulb, the two cuffs and the pressure release valve is determined by the position of the control lever. It can be seen that movements of the coarse and fine aneroid chambers are interactive by way of their linkage through the mechanism actuating the indicator on the read-out scale,[D] and Ponte J and Greene D, eds. 1986. A New Short Textbook of Anaesthetics, Edward Arnold, 1986.

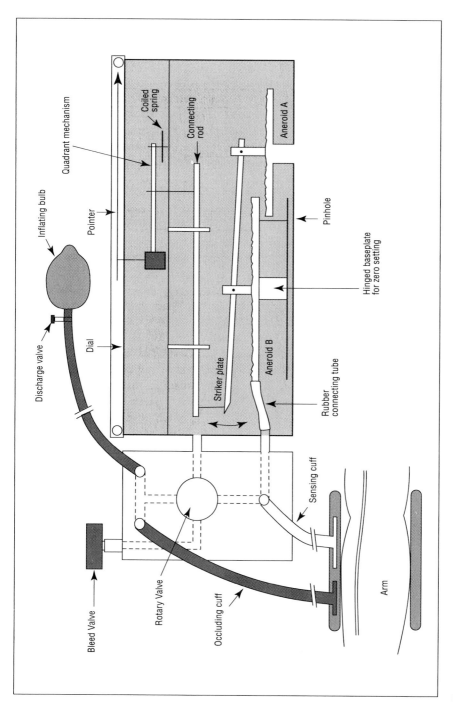

Figure 6.4 A diagrammatic cross-section through the oscillotonometer chamber, showing the manner in which the two aneroids interact through the fulcrum striker plate and the connecting rod and the additional provision for zero setting. The connections between inflating cuff, arm cuffs and bleed valve are again shown.[C]

which, when open, allows deflation of the occluding cuff but, when closed, ensures leak-free inflation.

Thus, in the inflation mode the interior of the instrument is pressurised and the pressure attained indicated on the dial. Because of the free communication which exists also between the inflating bulb and the two cuffs, these are increasingly pressurised with each squeeze of the bulb to the same pressure. As the diaphragm of the sensing cuff aneroid is subjected to the same pressure within and without, it exerts no additional influence on the mechanical output of the occluding cuff aneroid, so that the dial simply indicates the rising inflation pressure which, ultimately, will be raised to some 30 mm Hg above the expected systolic pressure by the operator.

When the bleed valve is opened to release the pressure in the occluding cuff, the pressure in that cuff, in the sensing cuff, and in the interior of the instrument falls accordingly, the inflating cuff now having been isolated from the system, whilst the two cuffs and the interior of the instrument remain in communication with one another.

As the pressure falls (as in the sphygmomanometric technique, it should be limited to <3 mm Hg/min for satisfactory results), the indicating pointer is seen to flick minimally in time with the heart beat, as the pulse strikes the upper margin of the occluding cuff and distorts it slightly. At this point, the sensing cuff plays no part, as no pulse can reach it.

With a further fall in the occlusive pressure, the energy in the blood during systole forces it past the previously occluding cuff. The corresponding pressure is shown on the dial but, superimposed on this is a small oscillation imparted by the aneroid connected to the sensing cuff, now distorted by the newly arriving pulse. There is some dispute concerning whether the first distinct change in the character of the oscillation or an abrupt change in amplitude of oscillation should be taken as denoting the initial release of occlusion of the artery.

As the pressure falls further, the pulsations become larger and correspondingly larger oscillations are conveyed from the sensing aneroid to the fulcrum plate, thereby enhancing the oscillation of the indicating pointer. It is at this point, where the oscillation undergoes a change in character, that the pressure in the occluding cuff may be taken as the systolic pressure.[17,18]

With continuing release of pressure, the indication corresponds to the degree of oscillation imparted to the sensing cuff around the indicated pressure still being applied to the artery by the occluding cuff, as it deflates. The ability of the sensing chamber to produce these valuable oscillations[19,20] is a function of the difference in size between the two cuffs and the different characteristics of the aneroid chambers.

As with sphygmomanometry, oscillotonometry is more reliable when the occluding cuff is deflated slowly and the reasons for this are essentially

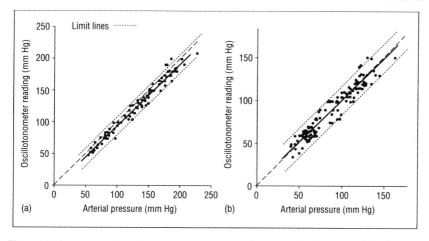

Figure 6.5 Comparison of oscillotonometer pressure determinations with direct arterial blood pressure recordings. The heavy line is the regression line and the dashed line is the line of identity. Fine dotted lines show the 95% confidence limits. It can be seen that with slow deflation of the cuff system (a) the limits are closer than those depicted when deflation is more rapid (b). Hence, the more rapid the deflation rate, the greater is the inaccuracy of the method.[A] *Cited as Br J Anaesth 1982;54:581–91.*

similar. However, experienced users, having determined the systolic pressure and having a reasonable expectation of the diastolic pressure being in a given range, in practice often increase the rate of deflation over the mid portion of the range between systolic and diastolic pressures, provided the displacement on the manometer dial remains substantial and shows no sign of decay. The readings over this part of the scale are ignored. A short pause is then allowed to ensure pressure equalisation. It is, of course, essential to set zero at the outset.

In a careful study, including comparison with direct arterial blood pressure readings, Hutton and Prys-Roberts[18] concluded that the end-point for determination of the diastolic pressure might not be clearly defined and, hence, could be partially subjective (Figure 6.5).

Potential problems

The performance of the oscillotonometer may be hampered by particles of dirt in the rotary and bleed valves or by their contamination by grease. The rate at which the system is deflated is critical, as too rapid a deflation leads to a disparity in pressure between that in the sensing cuff and that in the occluding cuff and the body of the instrument. The connection between the sensing cuff allows free passage of air, the intention being the maintenance of equilibrium between the sensing cuff and the rest of the pressurised parts of the system. However, the communication between the occluding cuff and the body of the instrument is more restrictive.

Sources of error

Since the principle involved is essentially that of sphygmomanometry, although the sensing mechanism is intimately bound to the occlusion apparatus, oscillotonometry suffers from the same deficiencies as sphygmomanometry. However, the principal advantages in use are:

- the sensitivity of the sensor;
- the relative clarity of the indication afforded by the pointer oscillations;
- the ability of the operator to view the pressure scale and the superimposed oscillations remote from the site of measurement, an important consideration in anaesthesia and certain critical care settings and also when repeated observations have to be made, as in surveillance monitoring.

Popularity and limitations

Until quite recently, the oscillotonometer has remained popular with anaesthetists. Its principal advantages were its portability and small size for accommodation close to patients. Since the patients are usually lying horizontally, the instrument is at or about the ideal level when placed beside them. Further, some volatile anaesthetic agents were prone to produce a degree of vasodilatation favourable to the instrument. It has, however, been less favoured by other groups of potential users.

Practical applications of oscillometry and oscillotonometry

The instruments in use today are firmly based on those designed by Von Recklinghausen. Although there are variations on the fundamental designs, that which has been in common use is the Scala Alternans Altera oscillotonometer.

Like all methods relying on the adequacy of perfusion for successful detection of the systolic pulse, oscillotonometry is most successful in vasodilated subjects and was used very satisfactorily in deliberate hypotension during general anaesthesia before the widespread use of direct

> ## Use of the oscillotonometer
>
> - The oscillotonometer is a delicate instrument. Treat it with care.
> - Remember that the cuff must be placed on the arm correctly (the oscillotonometer was designed as a bedside instrument). The tubing should leave the cuff in the direction of the patient's feet.
> - Always set or check zero calibration.
> - Slow deflation gives best results.
> - It is better than the sphygmomanometer in shock states but, if it is not reading clearly, consider intravascular monitoring.

intravascular blood pressure monitoring. It is correspondingly less satisfactory when patients are shocked, dehydrated and vasoconstricted.

The oscillotonometer is designed to be used at the bedside and anaesthetists need to remember that, when they are using it at the head of the operating table, the cuff still needs to be applied the correct way up, i.e. with the conducting tubing leaving the cuff system in the direction of the patient's feet. The tubing must be arranged to be free from kinks (which are not always visible when the tubing is under operating drapes), as reliable readings are dependent on undamped pressure transfer from cuff to oscillotonometer pressure-sensing chambers.

Correct placement of an appropriately sized cuff and its contained bladder in relation to the artery is important. It is important also that the cuff, when closely applied to the limb, is secured in such a manner that it cannot become loose or unravelled when inflated. Modern designs incorporating buckles, clasp, or Velcro bands are satisfactory.

The oscillotonometer is much less used now that automated blood pressure monitoring instruments are widely available. However, it is an instrument which should be remembered when the latter are not available or on those occasions when they fail.

Lastly, it should be remembered that it is a delicate precision instrument, despite its rugged external appearance, and it must be treated with due care.

Automated devices

In the early 1970s, a number of devices appeared as "blood pressure monitors" or "blood pressure followers". These used oscillometry or oscillotonometry and employed the pressure sensors of the period, where the amplified output was fed to digital displays. The systolic and diastolic values were achieved by sample-and-hold of the highest and lowest values.

The early machines were bulky and prone to artefact and had no effective artefact rejection.

In the later 1970s, the emergence of microprocessors, in particular the Intel 4004 in control applications, began to make an impact on medical equipment. The successor to the Intel 4004, the Intel 8080, was an advanced design for the period and its variant, the 8080A, was chosen for an automated blood pressure measurement apparatus based on oscillometry. The first "Dinamap"[21] (the name is an acronym representing Device for Indirect Non-invasive Automated Mean Arterial Pressure) displayed only the mean pressure, but had advantages over its predecessors in that, not only could repeated measurements be made, but faulty measurements could be detected and rejected before completion, and failed measurements re-attempted until acceptable to the device. However, users were generally unaccustomed to the mean pressure as an expression of arterial pressure and susceptibility to movement artefact was a significant problem.

Mean arterial pressure was selected for the first Dinamap as it was thought to indicate the effective driving pressure in the arterial system better than the systolic and diastolic pressures. It was also more robust as a measurement, in that it reflected the greatest amplitude of oscillations in the cuff. Two cuff hoses were used, even though it was accepted that one was sufficient, for operational reasons and for extra safety. One hose connected the cuff to the pressure sensor in the main unit, whilst the other was connected to the pumps, valves, and pressure limiting control. There were advantages in controlling inflation and deflation if more than one pneumatic circuit was used. Moreover, if either or both of the tubes was occluded, the pressure in the pneumatic sensing circuit was unchanged, so that the instrument could identify an external occlusion and alert the user. Cuff pressure was sensed by a solid-state pressure transducer and the signal processed by an amplifier and a by a microcomputer that also controlled the events of the device, including the characteristic stepped inflation pattern and the acceptance of pressures for output. Full details have been given by Ramsey.[22]

Critikon "Dinamap"

Refinement of the initial design and the production of algorithms capable of achieving substantial artefact rejection have nevertheless seen this type become the normal approach to blood pressure monitoring in recent years. Latterly, such microprocessor-based designs have been modified to provide certain derived information, as well as that obtained directly from the artery sensed, and they are often presented as modules in a complex monitoring array or as part of a clinical station, such as the anaesthesia workstation.

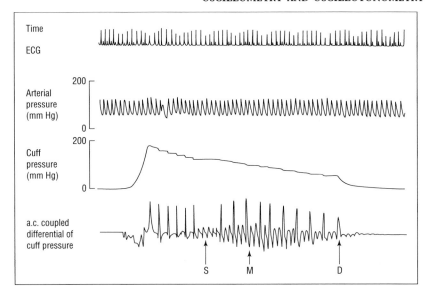

*Figure 6.6 Blood pressure estimation using the "Dinamap" compared with directly measured ipsilateral artery pressure. The lower trace shows the signal derived from cuff pressure oscillations, used by the "Dinamap" in determining systolic mean and diastolic enpoints,[A,C] and An assessment of the Dinamap 845, Anaesthesia; **39**:261–67. S = Systolic pressure, M = Mean pressure, D = Diastolic pressure.*

A typical trace is shown in Figure 6.6, and a block diagram of the Dinamap is shown in Figure 6.7.

Datex instrument

Another example is the Datex instrument (Figure 6.8), which is supplied free-standing or as a module in a modular assembly for use in anaesthesia, anaesthesia recovery and various types of critical care.

Importance of the deflation sequence

The deflation sequence of these instruments (Figure 6.9) merits special mention. It may be intermittent or continuous.

Intermittent

The term implies that the inflated cuff is allowed to deflate in steps. It follows that the size of the steps may be arbitrary in terms of a given application, since there is generally no provision for altering the magnitude

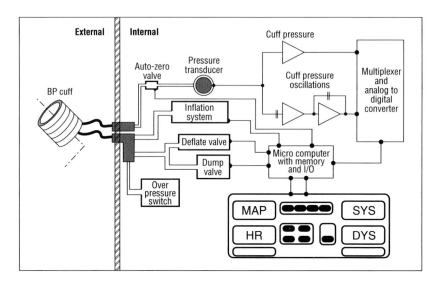

Figure 6.7 Diagrammatic representation of the Dinamap mechanism. Amplifiers are shown by the conventional symbols as are associated capacitors. Redrawn from[A] and Ramsey M 1991 J Clin Monit; 7:56–67. MAP=Mean arterial pressure; HR=Heart rate; SYS=Systolic blood pressure; DYS=Diastolic blood pressure.

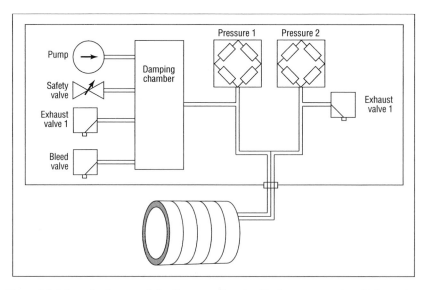

Figure 6.8 Schematic diagram of the Datex non-invasive blood pressure monitor. Redrawn from Instrumentarium Datex OY.

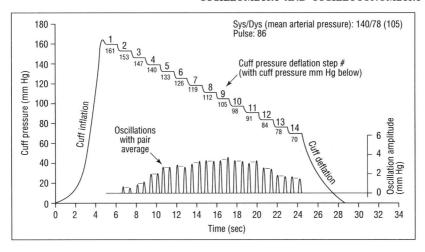

Figure 6.9 Cuff deflation sequence (Dinamap)[A].

of the steps. Each step change in pressure must then be maintained for sufficient time for a satisfactory estimation to be made. There is inevitably a trade-off between rapidity of descent (for rapid reading) and dwell time for the reading, and between rapidity of descent and the size of the drop in pressure (for accuracy of measurement). It is probably fair to say that, for many acute monitoring operations, users are uncritical of the values chosen by manufacturers for the step falls in pressure and the dwell time during which the device seeks to satisfy itself with the particular estimation. Users who need to be more critical, for example those tempted to use automated blood pressure monitors in hypertension follow-up or other systematic review (where accuracy is more important than short-term trend), may be less satisfied with such a random choice from their point of view. In these circumstances, small steps would be advantageous, whereas in anaesthesia or critical care, less accuracy might be balanced by speed and repetition capability.

Continuous

Some automated blood pressure monitors now permit continuous cuff deflation, whilst the pressure sensors associated with them send a continuous stream of digitised pressure information to the processor. An algorithm can determine whether the measurement is proceeding satisfactorily and can interrupt it if that is not the case. The digital feedback is especially useful in that it is possible for the device to discern usable waveforms and other characteristics of the flow in the artery under scrutiny.

95

> ## When using an automatic oscillometric blood pressure monitor*
>
> - Use a cuff of the correct size for the age of the patient.
> - Empty the cuff completely (by squeezing) before applying it to the patient.
> - Wrap it around the limb snuggly.
> - Keep the cuff about heart level.
> - If the reading does not seem reasonable, look at the patient and, conversely, ensure that a "malfunction" is not a clinical emergency.
> - In the event of suspected malfunction, check the cuff and hoses for leaks.
>
> * After Ramsey[21]

The major benefit here, apart from the obvious one of better artefact detection and rejection, is the possibility of recognising arrhythmias and similar disturbances which might be expected to interfere with readings but which should not necessarily provoke termination of a reading. A further advantage is a reduction in the number of read attempts after unsuccessful readings, thereby reducing the hazards associated with long periods of complete or partial vascular occlusion and, in the process, increasing the proportion of successful estimations, thereby increasing user satisfaction.

Many variants of the principle[22] have appeared as production instruments from a variety of manufacturers, and the serial method of making measurements has been validated.[23] Moreover, although many began as stand-alone devices, dedicated to blood pressure measurements and monitoring, they are increasingly incorporated into multifunction monitoring arrays suitable for use in the operating theatre, in coronary care, and intensive care units. Their very prevalence and the fact that they are automatic in much of their function is apt to lead users to disregard the need for the correct selection of cuffs[24] from available ranges, and their correct placement on the limb. Similarly, cuffs properly applied in the first instance may become dislodged in use, especially when out of sight, as in anaesthesia, and need to be checked or reapplied if their positioning has become unsatisfactory. It should also be noted that the results from these automated devices are subject to the same strictures on positioning of limbs and sensors as their non-automated counterparts.[25] Placing an infant cuff on the adult thumb is not a satisfactory arrangement.[26]

There is a tendency for blind faith to be placed in devices displaying numbers or traces and which are described as "electronic" or convey the notion that they are "computers". It is important that users are aware of

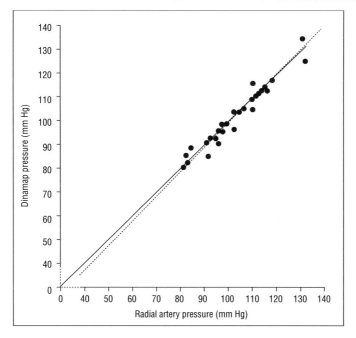

Figure 6.10 Relationship between systolic pressure measured by Dinamap monitor and that measured by radial artery catheter in infants and children. Redrawn from Park MK, and Menard SM. Accuracy of blood pressure measurement by the Dinamap monitor in infants and children, Pediatrics 1987;79:907–13.

the usual fallibility of such systems in the hands of human operators. The instructions should be read carefully, the instruments treated with respect, routine maintenance and calibration carried out according to the manufacturer's advice, and the output appreciated critically in the light of other clinical findings.

The performance of a number of these devices has been reviewed in the literature in the settings of adult,[18,27–51] paediatric, infant and neonatal (Figure 6.10),[52–61] emergency and transport[62] use, and in anaesthesia (Figure 6.11),[35,63–68] and intensive care.[69]

Portable and hand-held devices

Miniaturisation of electronic devices has been evident in the field of blood pressure monitors. Several Japanese manufacturers produced miniaturised devices during the early 1980s. Some of these have been reviewed by Johnson and Kerr.[70] It appeared that, despite their low cost when compared with the bench models, some of these devices performed very well and, in common with many Japanese hand-held calculators, incorporated miniature

97

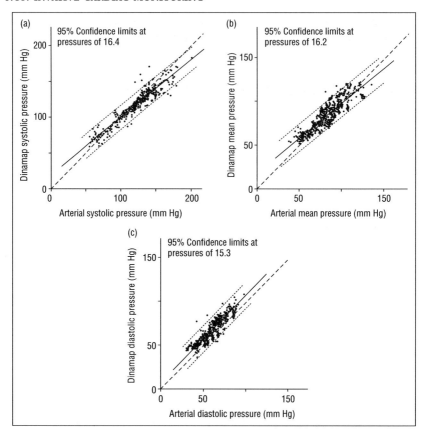

Figure 6.11 Comparison of Dinamap recordings with direct arterial blood pressure recordings. (a) Systolic pressure comparisons; (b) Mean pressure comparisons; (c) Diastolic pressure comparisons. The heavy lines are regression lines; dashed lines are lines of identity; light dotted lines represent 95% confidence limits at various pressures.[A] *Dye J and Hughes DG*, Anaesthesia 1987;**39**:261–67.

printers for hard-copy. In practice, despite these attractions, miniature automated blood pressure monitors have found little favour in the operating theatre and similar areas in hospitals. They have nevertheless been exploited to a limited extent in clinics and are increasingly used in primary care, in clinics and in the community, and also by patients and the public.

Evaluations

Detailed evaluations have been conducted in the UK by the Scientific and Technical Branch of the Department of Health (now the Medical Devices Agency, Hannibal House, Elephant & Castle, London, SE1 6TQ), in their *Health Equipment Information* (HEI) and *Evaluation* series, and in the USA by the Emergency Care Research Institute (ECRI).

Oscillometric monitoring in children and neonates

The cuff size is of special importance in neonates, infants, and small children.[56,57] Provided care is taken to avoid congestion and sustained vascular occlusion in limbs, the method has proved very effective for neonatal blood pressure monitoring.[55,58]

Accuracy and repeatability

Special problems arise in the evaluation of automated instruments.[71] Since the yardstick for blood pressure measurements remains intra-arterial measurement, it is salutary to look at the automated non-invasive method in comparison with direct measurement.

Several groups of workers have investigated the accuracy of automated blood pressure monitors in comparison with direct readings in adults,[18,35,68,72–74] and in children, infants and neonates.[56,59,75] The use of single or twin hoses does not appear to be important.[76]

Hazards of automated oscillometric techniques

Several hazards encountered with pressurised cuff devices and potentially occlusive sensors have been described.[77–79] A problem of particular importance in monitoring concerns the frequency of cuff inflations and is two-fold. First, repeated attempts may be made, especially by automated devices, to achieve a satisfactory reading when earlier readings have been thwarted by movement artefact, electrical interference, and similar interruptions. As the interval between attempts may be quite short, there may be insufficient time for satisfactory limb reperfusion after arterial occlusion, with consequent tissue damage,[67,80,81] including possible nerve damage.[82,83] Secondly, in an attempt to emulate near-continuous monitoring, the operator may be tempted to leave an insufficient interval between readings, with a similar outcome. The same error may prevent fluids being administered at the required rate,[84] or even at all, with serious consequences in the short term if the infusion is a vehicle for certain drugs. Some designs have incorporated a specific mode (sometimes called the "STAT" mode) which gives the user the opportunity to select a strictly limited period of frequent measurements to circumvent the problem.[85]

99

1 Von Recklinghausen H. Uber Blutdruckmessung beim Menschen. *Arch Exp Pathol Pharmakol* 1901; **46**: 78–132.
2 Howell WH, Brush CE. A critical note upon clinical methods of measuring blood pressure. *Boston Med Surg J* 1901; **145**: 146–51.
3 Erlanger J. A new instrument for determining the minimum and maximum blood pressure in man. *Johns Hopkins Hosp Rep* 1903; **12**: 53–100.
4 Sykes MK, Vickers MD. *Principles of measurement for anaesthetists.* Oxford: Blackwell Scientific Publications, 1970.
5 Hill DW. *Electronic techniques in medicine and surgery.* London: Butterworths, 1973.
6 Kleinman R. Understanding natural frequency and damping and how they relate to the measurement of blood pressure. *J Clin Monit* 1989; **5**: 137–47.
7 Bigliano RP, Molner SF, Sweeney LM. A new physiological pressure sensor. *Proc Ann Con Eng Med Biol* 1964; **6**: 82.
8 Pressman G, Newgard P. A transducer for continuous external measurement of blood pressure. *IEEE Trans Biomed Eng* 1963; **10**: 73–81.
9 Bahr DE, Ptezke JC. The automatic arterial tonometer. *Proc Ann Conf Eng Med Biol* 1973; **15**: 259.
10 Borkat FR, Kataoka RW, Silva J. An approach to the continuous non-invasive measurement of blood pressure. *Proc San Diego Biomed Symp* 1976.
11 Drzewiecki GM, Melbin J, Noordergraaf A. Arterial tonometry: review and analysis. *J Biomech* 1983; **16**: 141–52.
12 Eckerle JS. Tonometry, arterial. In: Webster JG ed. *Encyclopedia of medical devices and instrumentation.* New York: John Wiley and Sons, 1988.
13 Sato T, Nishinaga M, Kawamoto A, Ozawa T, Takatsuji H. Accuracy of a continuous blood pressure monitor based on arterial tonometry. *Hypertension* 1993; **21**: 866–74.
14 Stein PD, Blick EF. Arterial tonometry for the atraumatic measurement of arterial blood pressure. *J Appl Physiol* 1971; **31**: 593–6.
15 Von Recklinghausen H. *Neue Wege zur Blutdruckmessung.* Berlin: Springer Verlag, 1931.
16 Gallavardin L. Sur un nouveau brassard sphygmomanométrique. *Presse Médicale* 1922; **9**: 776.
17 Corrall IM, Strunin L. Assessment of the Von Recklinghausen oscillotonometer. *Anaesthesia* 1975; **30**: 59–66.
18 Hutton P, Prys-Roberts C. The oscillotonometer in theory and practice. *Br J Anaesth* 1982; **54**: 581–91.
19 Posey JA, Geddes LA, Williams H, Moore AG. The meaning of the point of maximum oscillations in cuff pressure in the indirect measurement of blood pressure. *Cardiovasc Res Center Bull* 1969; **8**: 15–25.
20 Mauck GW, Smith CR, Geddes LA, Bourland JD. The meaning of the point of maximum oscillations in cuff pressure in the indirect measurement of blood pressure. Part II. *Trans Am Soc Mech Eng J Biomed Eng* 1980; **102**: 28–33.
21 Ramsey M. Noninvasive automatic determination of mean arterial blood pressure. *Med Biol Eng Comput* 1979; **17**: 11–18.
22 Ramsey M. Blood pressure monitoring: automated oscillometric devices. *J Clin Monit* 1991; **6**: 56–67.
23 Slaby A, Josifko M. Does sequential automated measurement improve the estimate of resting blood pressure? *J Hum Hypertens* 1992; **6**: 31–4.
24 Goldthorp SL, Cameron A, Asbury AJ. Dinamap arm and thigh arterial pressure measurement. *Anaesthesia* 1986; **41**: 1032–5.
25 Kroeker EJ, Wood EH. Comparison of simultaneously recorded central and peripheral arterial pressure pulses during rest, exercise and tilted position in man. *Circ Res* 1955; **3**: 623–32.
26 Zornow MH, Schubert A, Todd MM. Intraoperative oscillometric arterial blood pressure monitoring using non-standard cuff locations. *Anesthesiology* 1986; **65**: A135.
27 Borrow KM, Newburger JM. Noninvasive estimate of central aortic pressure using the oscillometric method for analysing systemic artery pulsatile blood flow: comparative study of indirect systolic, diastolic, and mean brachial artery pressure with simultaneous direct ascending aortic pressure measurements. *Am Heart J* 1982; **103**: 879–86.

28 Silas JH, Barker AT, Ramsey LE. Clinical evaluation of Dinamap 845 automated blood pressure recorder. *Br Heart J* 1980; **43**: 202–5.

29 Morel D, Suter P. Étude d'une méthode automatique non-invasive de mesure de la pression artérielle systolique diastolique et moyen. *Annls Anesthesiol Franç* 1981; **22**: 61–6.

30 Whelton PK, Thompson SG, Barnes RG, Miall WE. Evaluation of the Vita-Stat automatic blood pressure recorder. A comparison with the random-zero sphygmomanometer. *Am J Epidemiol* 1983; **117**: 46–54.

31 Roy RC, Morgan L, Beamer D. Factitiously low blood pressure from the Dinamap. *Anesthesiology* 1983; **59**: 258–9.

32 Gloyna DF, Huber P, Abston P. A comparison of blood pressure measurement techniques in the hypotensive patient. *Anesth Analg* 1984; **63**: 222.

33 Van Egmond J, Hasenbros M, Crul JF. Invasive *v.* noninvasive blood pressure measurement of arterial pressure. *Br J Anaesth* 1985; **57**: 434–44.

34 Gourdeau M, Martin R, Lamarche Y, Tetreault L. Oscillometry and direct blood pressure: A comparative clinical study during deliberate hypotension. *Can Anaesth Soc J* 1986; **33**: 300–7.

35 Louber PG. Comparison of intra-arterial and automated oscillometric blood pressure measurement methods in postoperative hypertensive patients. *Med Instrum* 1986; **20**: 255–9.

36 Rutten AJ, Ilsley AH, Skowronski GA, Runciman WB. A comparative study of the measurement of mean arterial blood pressure using automatic oscillometers, arterial cannulation and auscultation. *Anaesth Intens Care* 1986; **14**: 58–65.

37 Gorback MS, Quill TJ. Comparison of two types of noninvasive blood pressure monitors. *Anesthesiology* 1988; **69**: A325.

38 Slaby A, Arenberger P, Josifko M, Hrabak P. Evaluation of automatic sphygmomano-meters. *Sb Lek* 1989; **91**: 274–84.

39 Van Egmond J, Hasenbos M, Crul JF. Invasive *v.* non-invasive measurement of arterial pressure. *Brit J Anaesth* 1989; **63**: 619–20P.

40 Rosner BA, Appel LJ, Raczynski JM *et al.* A comparison of two automated monitors in the measurement of blood pressure reactivity. Trials of Hypertension Prevention Collaborative Research Group. *Ann Epidemiol* 1990; **1**: 57–69.

41 Caramella JP, Hidou M, Claude E. Controlled trial of a non-invasive continuous blood pressure monitor: Cortronic AMP 770. *Annls Fr Anesth Reanim* 1991; **10**: 425–9.

42 Whincup PH, Bruce NG, Cook DG, Shaper AG. The Dinamap 1846X automated blood pressure recorder: comparison with the Hawksley random zero sphygmomanometer under field conditions. *J Epidemiol Commun Health* 1992; **46**: 164–9.

43 Amoore JN. Assessment of oscillometric non-invasive blood pressure monitors using the Dynatech Nevada CuffLink analyser. *J Med Eng Technol* 1993; **17**: 25–31.

44 Boaventura I, Fonseca T, Ramalhinho V, da Costa JN. Automatic measurement of arterial pressure. *Rev Port Cardiol* 1993; **12**: 133–9.

45 de Jong JR, Tepaske R, Scheffer GJ, Ros HH, Sipkema PP, de Lange JJ. Noninvasive continuous blood pressure measurement: a clinical evaluation of the Cortronic APM 770. *J Clin Monit* 1993; **9**: 18–24.

46 ECRI. Electronic, automatic sphygmomanometers. *J Healthcare Mater Manag* 1993; **11**: 44, 46, 48–57.

47 Marquez Contreras E, Martin de Pablos JL, Gutierrez Marin MC. Validation of an automatic noninvasive arterial pressure monitor: the ACP-2200. *Aten Primaria* 1994; **14**: 815–9.

48 Ng KG, Small CF. Survey of automated noninvasive blood pressure monitors. *J Clin Eng* 1994; **19**: 452–75.

49 Thummler M, Wonka F, Schoppe A. Preliminary clinical comparative study of a new blood pressure instrument with wrist cuff. *Z Kardiol* 1994; **83**: 641–5.

50 Ling J, Ohara Y, Orime Y, Noon GP, Takatani S. Clinical evaluation of the oscillometric blood pressure monitor in adults and children based on the 1992 AAMI SP-10 standards. *J Clin Monit* 1995 **11**: 123–30.

51 Ng K-G, Small CF. Survey of automated noninvasive blood pressure monitors. Published comments and errata. *J Clin Eng* 1995; **20**: 469–79.

101

52 Guntheroth WG, Nadas AS. Blood pressure measurements in infants and children. *Pediatr Clin N Amer* 1955; **2**: 257–63.

53 Sadove MS, Schmidt G, Wu HH, Katz D. Indirect blood pressure measurement in infants: a comparison of four methods in four limbs. *Anesth Analg* 1973; **52**: 682–9.

54 Dellagrammaticas HD, Wilson AJ. Clinical evaluation of the Dinamap non-invasive blood pressure monitor in pre-term neonates. *Clin Phys Physiol Meas* 1981; **2**: 271–6.

55 Friesen RH, Lichtor JL. Indirect measurement of blood pressure in neonates and infants utilising an automated non-invasive oscillometric monitor. *Anesth Analg* 1981; **60**: 742–5.

56 Kimble KJ, Darnell RA, Yelderman M, Araigno RL, Ream AK. An automated oscillometric technique for estimating mean arterial blood pressure in critically ill newborns. *Anesthesiology* 1981; **54**: 423–5.

57 Pellegrini-Caliumi G, Agostino R, Dodari S, Meffe G, Morett C, Bucci E. Evaluation of an automated oscillometric method and various cuffs for the measurement of arterial blood pressure in the neonate. *Acta Paediatr Scand* 1982; **71**: 791–7.

58 Cullen PM, Dye J, Hughes DG. Clinical assessment of the neonatal Dinamap 847. *J Clin Monit* 1987; **3**: 229–34.

59 Park MK, Menard SM. Accuracy of blood pressure measurement by the Dinamap monitor in infants and children. *Pediatrics* 1987; **79**: 907–13.

60 Park MK, Guntheroth WG. Accurate blood pressure measurement in children. *Am J Non-invasive Cardiol* 1989; **3**: 297–309.

61 Weaver MG, Park MK, Lee DH. Differences in blood pressure levels obtained by auscultatory and oscillometric methods. *Am J Dis Child* 1990; **144**: 911–14.

62 Runcie CJ, Reeve WG, Reidy J, Dougall JR. Blood pressure measurement during transport. A comparison of direct and oscillometric readings in critically ill patients. *Anaesthesia* 1990; **45**: 659–65.

63 Yelderman M, Ream AK. A microprocessor based automated non-invasive blood pressure device for the anesthetised patient. In: Martin JI ed. *Proc San Diego Biomed Symp 17*. New York: Academic Press, 1977.

64 Yelderman M, Ream AK. Indirect measurement of mean blood pressure on the anaesthetized patient. *Anesthesiology* 1979; **50**: 253–6.

65 Hutton P, Dye J, Prys-Roberts C. An assessment of the Dinamap 845. *Anaesthesia* 1982; **39**: 261–7.

66 Moyle JTB. Non-invasive monitoring in anaesthesia. In: Kaufman L ed. *Anaesthesia Review 11*. Edinburgh: Churchill Livingstone, 1984.

67 De Silva PHDP, Mostafa SM. Assessment of Dinamap 845. *Anaesthesia* 1985; **40**: 817.

68 Nystrom E, Reid KH, Bennett R, Couture L, Edmonds HL Jr. A comparison of automated indirect arterial blood pressure meters: with recordings from a radial artery catheter in anesthetized surgical patients. *Anesthesiology* 1985; **62**: 526–30.

69 Frucht U *et al.* How reliable are indirect blood pressure measurement devices in the intensive care unit (ICU)? In: Meyer-Sabellek W *et al.* eds. *Blood pressure measurements*. New York: Springer-Verlag, 1990.

70 Johnson CJM, Kerr JM. Automatic blood pressure monitors. A clinical evaluation of five models in adults. *Anaesthesia* 1985; **40**: 471–8.

71 Appel LJ, Marwaha S, Whelton PK, Patel M. The impact of automated blood pressure devices on the efficiency of clinical trials. *Controlled Clin Trials* 1992; **13**: 240–7.

72 Sapinski A, Szuman J, Jasinski J. Measurement of arterial blood pressure using the sphygmomanometer-S and the direct method. *Kardiol Pol* 1991; **35**: 174–6.

73 Papadopoulos G, Oldorp B, Mieke S. Arterial blood pressure measurement with oscillometric instruments in newborns and infants. *Anaesthesist* 1994; **43**: 441–6.

74 Rithalia SV, Edwards D. Comparison of oscillometric and intra-arterial blood pressure and pulse measurement. *J Med Eng Technol* 1994; **18**: 179–81.

75 Ramsey M 3d. Automatic oscillometric NIBP (noninvasive automatic blood pressure machines) versus manual auscultatory blood pressure in the PACU. *J Clin Monit* 1994; **10**: 136–9.

76 Amoore JN, Scott DH. Noninvasive blood pressure measurements with single and twin-hose systems – do mixtures matter? *Anaesthesia* 1993; **48**: 799–802.

77 Showman A, Betts EK. Hazards of automatic noninvasive blood pressure monitoring. *Anesthesiology* 1981; **55**: 717–8.

78 Bause GS, Weintraub AC, Tanner GE. Skin avulsion during oscillometry. *J Clin Monit* 1986; **2**: 262–3.
79 Celoria G, Dawson JA, Teres, D. Compartment syndrome in a patient monitored with an automated pressure cuff. *J Clin Monit* 1987; **3**: 139–41.
80 Nicholls BJ, Ryan DW. Petechial rashes and automatic blood pressure measurement. *Anaesthesia* 1986; **41**: 88.
81 Vidal P, Sykes PJ, O'Shaughnessy M, Craddock K. Compartment syndrome after use of an automatic arterial pressure monitoring device. *Br J Anaesth* 1993; **71**: 902–4 (An erratum appears in *Br J Anaesth* 1994; **72**: 738).
82 Sy WP. Ulnar nerve palsy possibly related to use of automatically cycled blood pressure cuff. *Anesth Analg* 1981; **60**: 687–8.
83 Bickler OE, Schapera A, Bainton CR. Acute radial nerve injury from use of an automatic blood pressure monitor. *Anesthesiology* 1990; **73**: 186–8.
84 Brin EN, Lewis TC, Brin JA. A simple method for reducing backup of blood into intravenous lines caused by inflation of a blood pressure cuff. *Anesth Analg* 1990; **71**: 569.
85 Block FE, Fletcher MV, Morris TJ, Dzwonczyk R. A clinical evaluation of rapid automatic non-invasive blood pressure determination with the Ohmeda 2120 "return to flow" method. *J Clin Monit* 1991; 7: 241–4.

7 The force-balance principle and related methods of tonometry

Penaz in 1973 coined the term "the unloaded artery principle" to denote his method of exploiting the force-balance principle.[1-7] This embodies the notion that any force exerted by a body may be opposed by an equivalent (known or measurable) force in order to establish its magnitude. The attraction of the principle in monitoring lies in the fact that known or easily measured opposing forces are used and the sole requirement is to achieve a null balance between the forces, known and unknown, and establish that is the case.[8]

The apparatus needed comprises a cuff which is capable of rapid inflation-deflation and a photoelectric detection system (Figure 7.1). In practice, the cuff is alternately inflated and deflated by an electronic control system

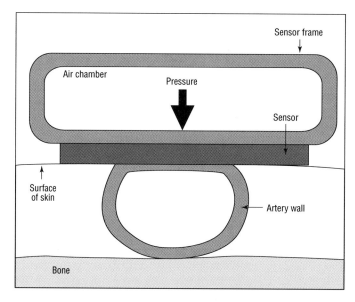

Figure 7.1 Diagram showing the principle of arterial tonometry. The artery is partially flattened between the sensor and the underlying bone. The sensor contains piezo-resistive pressure transducers. Redrawn from Kemmotsu et al., Anesthesiology 1991;75:333–40.

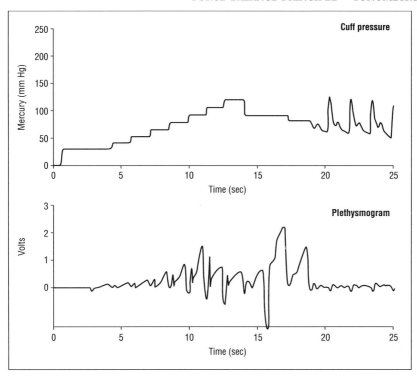

Figure 7.2 Penaz principle applied to the finger. The finger blood pressure monitor increases pressure in the finger cuff incrementally (top trace) and analyses the resultant plethysmogram (bottom trace) at each increment to determine the artery size when transmitted pressure equals 0 (unloaded artery). Once this point is determined, the artery is kept at that unloaded size by controlling the pressure in the cuff,[B] and Boehmer RD, Continuous real-time non-invasive monitor of blood pressure, Penaz methodology applied to the finger J Clin Monit 1987;3:282–87.

and sensing is by means of a source of light (usually a light emitting diode and a photo-cell sensor). Since the sensing system detects optical density it is, by extrapolation, sensing change in volume and is thus an effective plethysmograph. The fact that it is poor at estimating the actual volume is irrelevant in the context. The control system employs feedback in order to correct the pressure in the finger cuff sufficiently rapidly and frequently to maintain the optical signal seen by the photosensor to remain constant in practical terms. The feedback signal itself thus represents the extent of correction being applied and, hence, the oscillating signal corresponding to the pulsation in the proximal feeding artery (Figure 7.2).

Instruments using the force-balance principle as implemented here and commercially represented by the Ohmeda *Finapres* instrument[9,10] may be expected to be subject to the same limitations as those operating on the other principles already described and which rely on good perfusion and sufficient vascular flexibility for successful clinical exploitation. Sources of error have been identified,[11] as have other factors affecting the performance and reliability of such devices.[12]

The finger cuff is of low volume and is non-distensible, in order that it may respond sufficiently rapidly to the signals received from the transillumination pair comprising a photo diode transmitting infrared light at a wavelength of 925 nm and a photo-cell receiver. However, the response of the system is also limited by the delays inherent in the admission and release of pressurised air to and from the cuff. The mean pressure is sensed first, whereupon the instrument then responds to the changes in optical density to follow the changes in blood pressure at a level where the oscillation is detected as maximal. However, even during tachycardia, the instrument is sufficiently sensitive and rapidly responding to be clinically useful. Not surprisingly, in view of the operating principle, the device performs best when the local blood vessels are dilated.[13]

Early experience created a favourable impression,[14] confirming non-clinical studies already carried out.[15] Although there have been arguments about the merits of the device in adults on the basis of comparisons with direct arterial pressure measurements,[12,13,16–20] it has proved valuable in small children, infants and neonates in whom other methods of measurement are difficult. Moreover, it has the advantage of providing near-continuous beat-by-beat measurement of the blood pressure with a much reduced risk of occlusion injury, although this latter is not unknown.[21] A detailed review of comparative results from a number of workers is given by Hutton and Clutton-Brock[22] (Figure 7.3).

Clinical application

Clinically, the Finapres appears to have been well received when used in relatively undemanding applications, such as the monitoring of patients on CPAP[23] or in circumstances where direct arterial monitoring was neither possible nor desirable or alternative methods were not superior.[24–26] In uncomplicated anaesthesia the device seems have to have been regarded as acceptable,[27] provided continuous monitoring was not essential,[20,28] although the early cuff design was thought to need improvement[29] and dislodgement of the cuff was seen to be a problem.[30] An interesting study showed the Finapres to be competent in estimation of the aortic pressure during cardiac catheterisation.[31]

More demanding circumstances have revealed some shortcomings.[32,33] In obstetric practice, the Finapres was considered to give results comparable with those obtained by oscillometric means, but the overall performance in that setting was found wanting.[26] During controlled hypotension under general anaesthesia, the blood pressure monitoring by tonometry was considered satisfactory,[34] but was less satisfactory in profound hypotension

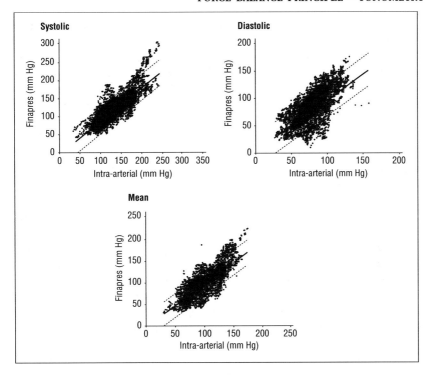

Figure 7.3 Comparison of measurements of systolic, diastolic and mean arterial blood pressure by Finapres with intra-arterial readings,[Δ] and Stokes DN et al., Br J Anaesth *1991;67:26–35.*

where it was stated that direct arterial monitoring was preferable;[35] it was also thought unsuitable for monitoring the blood pressure during the induction of anaesthesia preceding neurosurgery.[18] Although the Finapres has been used during one-lung anaesthesia for thoracic surgery, it tended to underestimate the blood pressure in normal two-lung anaesthesia and overestimate it during one-lung anaesthesia. It was recommended that direct arterial monitoring be used in these circumstances.[36] During and after cardiac bypass, it was found that satisfactory readings could not always be obtained.[37] It has also been used in the care of the critically ill,[38] although the investigators did not consider it a replacement for the conventional monitoring techniques. The Finapres has been reported as having been used successfully in the monitoring of autonomic dysfunction.[39] Although this type of finger tonometer was formerly unsatisfactory during bicycle ergometry,[17] it was thought to have a place in ambulatory blood pressure monitoring.[40] A new device, the *Portapres*, similar in concept to the Finapres, has been introduced and its suitability for ambulatory blood pressure monitoring confirmed.[41] It has been recommended for 24-hour ambulatory monitoring.[42]

In addition to the foregoing, other studies and evaluations have been conducted.[43-49] Tonometric devices similar to the Finapres have also been evaluated.[50-52]

More recently, the value of tonometry in the monitoring of children undergoing general anaesthesia has been confirmed,[53,54] but the Finapres could not be recommended for use in obstetric anaesthesia and analgesia.[55] Tonometry has been compared with direct arterial measurement,[56] and the principle has again been examined and described succinctly[57] as a prelude to the clinical use of the N-CAT tonometer,[58] which has been evaluated.[56] It seems that there are some limitations in practice.[58] Another new design is the *Vasotrac* tonometer system.[59]

Despite the demanding technique required, ultrasound detection of the blood pressure may be very satisfactory when proper care is taken. Hence, in circumstances where the subject can be encouraged to be quite still or is unconscious during the measurement, good results may be expected.

Despite the acknowledged drawbacks of the technique, these must be set against the potential hazards of radial artery cannulation.[60-62] Nevertheless, the intermittent nature of the recordings (in the case of all but the continuous plethysmographs) and, in some cases, the relatively poor correlation with intravascular pressure readings, militates against their general adoption in critical care and in some anaesthetic subspecialities, when an arterial line may be required in any case for other purposes.

Pulse oximetry in blood pressure monitoring by tonometry/plethysmography

The ability of the pulse oximeter to detect oxygenated blood has prompted its use as a detector in blood pressure estimation. It suffers from some specific disadvantages, in that it relies in the first instance on a satisfactory level of haemoglobin and suffers from the usual forms of interference.[63,64] It is also necessary to avoid spurious reinflation of the associated occluding cuff when inflation above the systolic level causes loss of the expected signal.[65] Given good operating conditions, however, performance is on a par with that of other indirect methods of blood pressure measurement. Like the force-balance method, it is easier to apply to children, infants and neonates than the more generally popular indirect methods. Comparisons have been made with other techniques of blood pressure measurement,[65,66] whilst pulse oximetry has been used for blood pressure assessment in pulseless disease.[67]

1 Penaz J. Photoelectric measurement of blood pressure, flow and volume in the finger. In: Roald A, ed. *Digest of the 10th International conference of medical and biological engineering.* Dresden: The International Federation of Medical and Biological Engineering, 1973.

2 Yamakoshi K, Shimazu H, Shibata M, Kamiya A. A new oscillometric method for indirect measurement of systolic and mean arterial pressure in the human finger. Part 2: Correlation study. *Med Biol Eng Comput* 1982; **20**: 314–18.

3 Drzewiecki GM, Melbin J, Noordergraaf A. Arterial tonometry: review and analysis. *J. Biomech* 1983; **16**: 141–52.

4 Molhoek GP, Wesseling KH, Settels JJM. Evaluation of the Penaz servoplethysmomanometer for continuous non-invasive measurement of finger blood pressure. *Basic Res Cardiol* 1984; **79**: 598–609.

5 Wesseling KH, Settels JJ, De Wit B. The measurement of continuous finger arterial pressure non-invasively in stationary subjects. In: Schmidt TH, Dembrowski TM, Blumchen G, eds. *Biological and social factors in cardiovascular disease*. Berlin: Springer-Verlag, 1986: 355–75.

6 Rossberg F, Penaz J. The current status of noninvasive blood pressure measurement technics. *Z Gesamte Inn Med* 1989; **44**: 437–41.

7 Kemmotsu O, Ueda M, Otsuka H, Yamamura T, Winter D, Eckerle JS. Arterial tonometry for non-invasive, continuous blood pressure monitoring during anesthesia. *Anesthesiology* 1991; **75**: 333–40.

8 Shirer HW. Blood pressure measuring methods. *IRE Trans Biomed Eng* 1962; **9**: 116–25.

9 Hartmann B, Bassenge E. Noninvasive, continuous measurement of finger artery pressure with the servo-plethysmo-manometer Finapres. *Herz* 1989; **14**: 251–9.

10 Boehmer RD. Continuous, real-time, non-invasive monitor of blood pressure: Penaz methodology applied to the finger. *J Clin Monit* 1987; **3**: 282–7.

11 Kobler H, Cejnar M, Hunyor SN. Relevance of the waterfall phenomenon in continuous finger cuff blood pressure measurements. *Clin Exp Pharmacol Physiol* 1991; **18**: 323–6.

12 Kurki T, Smith NT, Head N, Dec-Silver H, Quinn A. Noninvasive continuous blood pressure measurement from the finger: optimal measurement conditions and factors affecting reliability. *J Clin Monit* 1987; **3**: 6–13.

13 Peschel SM, Melendez JA, Wald A, Weissman C. Noninvasive continuous blood pressure monitoring during sodium nitroprusside induced hypotension. *Anesthesiology* 1988; **69** (Suppl. 3A): A322.

14 Pasch T. Measurement of blood pressure during the intraoperative period. *Ann Fr Anesth Reanim* 1989; **8**: 532–5, 572–5.

15 Bos WJ, Imholz BP, van Goudoever J, Wesseling KH, van Montfrans GA. The reliability of noninvasive continuous finger blood pressure measurement in patients with both hypertension and vascular disease. *Amer J Hypertens* 1992; **5**: 529–35.

16 Smith NT, Wesseling KH, deWit B. Evaluation of two prototype devices producing noninvasive, pulsatile, calibrated blood pressure measurement from a finger. *J Clin Monit* 1985; **1**: 17–29.

17 Idema RN, van den Meiracker AH, Imholz BP *et al.* Comparison of Finapres non-invasive beat-to-beat finger blood pressure with intrabrachial artery pressure during and after bicycle ergometry. *J Hypertens* 1989; **7** (Suppl.): S58–9.

18 Kermode JL, Davis NJ, Thompson WR. Comparison of the Finapres blood pressure monitor with intra-arterial manometry during induction of anaesthesia. *Anaesth Intens Care* 1989; **17**: 470–5.

19 Parati G, Casadei R, Gropelli A, De Rienzo M, Mancia G. Comparison of finger and intra-arterial blood pressure monitoring at rest and during laboratory testing. *Hypertension* 1989; **13**: 647–55.

20 Stokes DN, Clutton-Brock T, Patil C, Thompson JM, Hutton P. Comparison of invasive and non-invasive measurements of continuous arterial pressure using the Finapres. *Brit J Anaesth* 1991; **67**: 26–35.

21 Gravenstein JS, Paulus DA, Feldman JM, McLaughlin G. Tissue hypoxia distal to a Penaz finger blood pressure cuff. *J Clin Monit* 1985; **2**: 120–5.

22 Hutton P, Clutton-Brock TH. The non-invasive measurement of blood pressure. In: Hutton P, Prys-Roberts C, eds. *Monitoring in anaesthesia and intensive care*. London: WB Sanders Co, 1994: 115–16.

23 Sforza E, Capecchi V, Lugaresi E. Haemodynamic effects of short-term nasal continuous positive airway pressure therapy in sleep apnoea syndrome: monitoring by a finger arterial pressure device. *Eur Respir J* 1992; **5**: 858–63.

24 Epstein RH, Kaplan S, Leighton BL, Norris MC, De Simone CA. Evaluation of continuous noninvasive blood pressure monitor in obstetric patients undergoing spinal anesthesia. *J Clin Monit* 1989; **5**: 157–63.

25 Epstein RH, Bartkowski RR, Huffnagle S. Continuous non-invasive finger blood pressure during controlled hypotension. A comparison with intraarterial pressure. *Anesthesiology* 1991; **75**: 796–803.

26 Porter KB, O'Brien WF, Kiefert V, Knuppel RA. Finapres: a noninvasive device to monitor blood pressure. *Obstet Gynecol* 1991; **78**: 430–3.

27 Kemmotsu O, Ueda M, Otsuka H, Yamamura T, Winter DC, Eckerle JS. Arterial tonometry for noninvasive, continuous blood pressure monitoring during anesthesia. *Anesthesiology* 1991; **75**: 333–40.

28 Gibbs NM, Larach DR, Derr JA. The accuracy of Finapres noninvasive mean arterial pressure measurements in anesthetized patients. *Anesthesiology* 1991; **74**: 647–52.

29 Schiller Z, Pasch T. Servo-plethysmo-manometry for continuous noninvasive blood pressure monitoring. *Anaesthesist* 1991; **40**: 105–9.

30 Jones RD, Kornberg JP, Roulson CJ, Visram AR, Irwin MG. The Finapres 2300e finger cuff. The influence of cuff application on the accuracy of blood pressure measurement. *Anaesthesia* 1993; **48**: 611–15.

31 Virolainen J. Use of non-invasive finger blood pressure monitoring in the estimation of aortic pressure at rest and during the Mueller manoeuvre. *Clin Physiol* 1992; **12**: 619–28.

32 Epstein RH, Bartowski RR. Evaluation of a continuous non-invasive blood pressure monitor during deliberate hypotension in orthopedic patients. *Anesthesiology* 1988; **69** (Suppl. 3A): A323.

33 Gibbs NM, Larach DR, Derr JA. The performance of the FINAPRES continuous blood pressure monitor during the peri-induction period in high-risk patients. *Anesthesiology* 1988; **69**: A324.

34 Kemmotsu O, Ueda M, Otsuka H *et al.* Blood pressure measurement by arterial tonometry in controlled hypotension. *Anesth Analg* 1991; **73**: 54–8.

35 Aitken HA, Todd JG, Kenny GNC. Comparison of the Finapres and direct arterial pressure monitoring during profound hypotensive anaesthesia. *Brit J Anaesth* 1991; **67**: 36–40.

36 Bardoczky GI, Levarlet M, Engelman E, d'Hollander A, Schmartz D. Continuous noninvasive blood pressure monitoring during thoracic surgery. *J Cardiothorac Vasc Anesth* 1992; **6**: 51–4.

37 Kurki TS, Smith NT, Sanford TJ, Head N. Pulse oximetry and finger blood pressure measurement during open heart surgery. *J Clin Monit* 1989; **5**: 221–8.

38 Farquhar IK. Continuous direct and indirect blood pressure measurement (Finapres) in the critically ill. *Anaesthesia* 1991; **46**: 1050–5.

39 Tanaka H, Thulesius O, Yamaguchi H, Mino M. Circulatory responses in children with unexplained syncope evaluated by continuous non-invasive finger blood pressure monitoring. *Acta Paediatr* 1994; **83**: 754–61.

40 Kawarada A, Shimazu H, Ito H, Yamakoshi K. Ambulatory monitoring of indirect beat-to-beat arterial pressure in human fingers by a volume-compensation method. *Med Biol Eng Comput* 1991; **29**: 55–62.

41 Schmidt TF, Wittenhaus J, Steinmetz TF, Piccolo P, Lupsen H. Twenty-four-hour ambulatory noninvasive continuous finger blood pressure measurement with PORTAPRES: a new tool in cardiovascular research. *J Cardiovasc Pharmacol* 1992; **19** (Suppl. 6): S117–45.

42 Imholz BP, Langewouters GJ, van Montfrans GA *et al.* Feasibility of ambulatory, continuous 24-hour finger arterial pressure recording. *Hypertension* 1993; **21**: 65–73.

43 Dorlas JC, Nuboer JA, Butijn WT, Var der Hoeven GM, Settels JJ, Wesseling KH. Effects of peripheral vaso-constriction on the blood pressure in the finger, measured continuously by a new non-invasive method (the Finapres). *Anesthesiology* 1985; **62**: 342–5.

44 Imholz BPM, van Montfrans GA, Settels JJ, van der Hoeven GMA, Karemaker JM, Weiling W. Continuous non-invasive blood pressure monitoring: reliability of Finapres device during Valsalva manoeuvre. *Cardiovasc Res* 1988; **22**: 390–7.

45 Gorback MS, Quill TJ, Bloch EC, Graubert D. Oscillometric blood pressure determination from the adult thumb using an infant cuff. *Anesth Analg* 1989; **69**: 668–70.

46 Lamantia KR, O'Connor T, Barash PG. Comparing methods of measurement: an alternative approach. *Anesthesiology* 1990; **72**: 781–3.

47 Mulder LJM, Veldman JBP, Rüddel H, Robbe HWJ, Mulder G. On the usefulness of finger-pressure measurements for studies on mental workload. *Homeostasis* 1991; **33**: 47–60.

48 Imholz BMP, Parati G, Mancia G, Wesseling KH. Effects of graded vasoconstriction upon the measurement of finger arterial pressure. *J Hypertens* 1992; **10**: 979–84.

49 O'Brien E, Atkins N. Blood pressure measurement using oscillometric finger cuffs. *Anaesthesia* 1995; **50**: 743–5.

50 Wong DT, Volgyesi GA, Bissonnette B. Systolic arterial pressure determination by a new pulse monitor technique. *Can J Anaesth* 1992; **39**: 596–9.

51 Latman NS. Evaluation of finger blood pressure monitoring instruments. *Biomed Instrum Technol* 1992; **26**: 52–7.

52 Veerman DP, Lenders JW, Thien T, van Montfrans GA. LAM 100/Marshall F-88: accuracy and precision of a new device for discontinuous finger blood pressure measurement. *J Hum Hypertens* 1993; 7: 113–15.

53 Kemmotsu O. Noninvasive, continuous blood pressure measurement by arterial tonometry during anesthesia in children. *Anesthesiology* 1994; **81**: 1162–8.

54 Lyew MA, Jamieson JW. Blood pressure measurement using oscillometric finger cuffs in children and young adults. A comparison with arm cuffs during general anaesthesia. *Anaesthesia* 1994; **49**: 895–9.

55 Wilkes MP, Bennett A, Hall P, Lewis M, Clutton-Brock TH. Comparison of invasive and non-invasive measurement of continuous arterial pressure using the Finapres in patients undergoing spinal anaesthesia for lower segment caesarean section. *Brit J Anaesth* 1994; **73**: 738–43.

56 Siegel LC, Brock-Utne JG, Brodsky JB. Comparison of arterial tonometry with radial artery catheter measurements of blood pressure in anesthetized patients. *Anesthesiology* 1994; **81**: 578–84.

57 Searle NR, Gauthier J, Sahab P. An evaluation of the N-CAT, a new arterial tonometer. *Can J Anaesth* 1995; **42**: 526–31.

58 Searle NR, Perrault J, Ste-Marie H, Dupont C. Assessment of the arterial tonometer (N-CAT) for the continuous blood pressure measurement in rapid atrial fibrillation. *Can J Anaesth* 1993; **40**: 388–93.

59 Belani KG, Buckley JJ. The new Vasotrac™ system – a novel continual noninvasive blood pressure monitor. *Anesthesiology* 1995; **83**: A489.

60 Bedford RF, Wollman H. Complications of per-cutaneous radial-artery cannulation; an objective prospective study in man. *Anesthesiology* 1973; **38**: 226–36.

61 Mangano DT, Hickey RF. Ischemic injury following uncomplicated radial artery cannulation. *Anesth Analg* 1979; **58**: 55–7.

62 Slogoff S, Keats AS, Arlund C. On the safety of radial artery cannulation. *Anesthesiology* 1983; **59**: 42–7.

63 Moyle JBT. *Pulse oximetry.* London: BMJ Publishing Group, 1994.

64 Hanning CD, Alexander-Williams JM. Pulse oximetry: a practical review. *BMJ* 1995; **311**: 367–70.

65 Wallace CT, Baker JD, Alpert CC, Tankersley SJ, Conroy JM, Kerns RE. Comparison of blood pressure measurements by doppler and by pulse oximetry techniques. *Anesth Analg* 1987; **66**: 1018–19.

66 Talke P, Nichols RJ, Traber DL. Does measurement of systemic blood pressure with a pulse oximeter correlate with conventional methods? *J Clin Monit* 1990; **6**: 5–9.

67 Chawla R, Kumarrel V, Girdhark KK, Sethi AK, Battacharya A. Oximetry in pulseless disease. *Anaesthesia* 1990; **45**: 992–3.

8 Problems and errors in blood pressure measurement and instrumentation

It is pertinent to discuss some of the difficulties that arise when methods of determining blood pressure are assessed or compared.[1] Quite apart from any problems associated with the design and construction of the devices themselves,[2,3] matters concerning observer errors and bias[4-7] and other aspects of statistical comparison[8] must be considered, as must the conditions under which studies are conducted in this field.[9] Good examples are to be found in the sometimes heated debate surrounding the establishment of zero and the elimination of errors arising from it in sphygmomanometric measurements[10-15] and the measures taken to help overcome the difficulties.[16,17] In addition, it is easy to assume that we instinctively know what it is we expect from a monitoring device or system, based on assumptions that we may make about the discipline to which monitoring is being applied. This is not necessarily so and needs careful consideration.[18]

A result of the foregoing is that workers in the field may take independent approaches to techniques of measurement.[19,20] One solution is to attempt to standardise the methods of measurement[21-23] or the instrument.[24] Blood pressure monitoring also introduces a potential source of predictive error in that the circumstances of having the blood pressure measurement taken may influence its level at the time,[25] a benign phenomenon which has become known as "white coat hypertension".[26-28]

The problems are sufficiently serious in the case of assessing blood pressure measuring instruments for protocols to have been devised for this purpose.[29-39] However, differences of opinion and interpretation exist concerning the protocols.[40]

Common sources of clinical error

Observer error

Observer error is a complex topic, but concerns the manner in which the person making the blood pressure measurement interprets the reading when this is not predetermined or fixed (as in the case of some automated devices). For example, the observer may have certain preconceptions about what he or she believes the value should or might be as the mercury column falls or the pointer oscillates. It has been amply demonstrated that such preconceptions influence the observer in selecting the point at which the pressure is recorded. We refer to this and similar aberrations on the part of the observer as *observer bias*.

When the measurement takes some time to perform, there is a temptation to *accelerate the process* in the belief that the first values perceived will in any case be correct.

When a mercury column or a pointer is moving, it is difficult to determine where the movement is centred or, if unidirectional, where to establish the *point of the reading*. This is complicated by the fact that there is almost always *visible oscillation* of the mercury column or the aneroid or the pointer caused simply by the small movement of the cuff as the pulse strikes it during occlusion.

To what *accuracy* should the observer read under these circumstances? Many records reveal that the blood pressure is annotated in steps of 2 or perhaps 5 mm Hg. Do we read to the nearest 5 above or below?

In the case of a pointer, viewing from positions other than perpendicular to the dial may produce appreciable *parallax* errors. A similar, though less obvious error may result if the mercury column is viewed from a position significantly above or below the level of the meniscus.

In short, the mental stratagems of the observer, combined with the intrinsic errors and practical problems of the methods make it probable that monitoring of blood pressure is often influenced in such ways. We need to be aware of the fact when making observations. They are likely to encourage us to take more care in their performance.

A more insidious error concerns the *transfer of observed results* to paper when recording or charting is not automatic. Again, there is good evidence that results having an unfavourable trend may be "rounded up" when committed to permanency. The same treatment may be afforded transient, though significant movements, or they may simply be omitted from the record. This "*smoothing*" of records and the appreciation by authorities of its prevalence is one of the driving forces behind the tendency towards requiring hard-copy records in certain clinical circumstances.

Zero errors

Any instrument whose results are referable to a zero baseline must be automatically zeroed or capable of having zero set and checked.

In the case of aneroid gauges, this is not always so, in which case they must be checked from time to time. Otherwise, the user should make it a

---

Some general sources of error in blood pressure monitoring and measurement

Design, construction and maintenance

- Poor design or manufacture
- Breakage (may be unseen in the case of glass tubes)
- Leaks (in glass, tubing, bulb, or the bellows of aneroid devices)
- Mercury leaks and consequent loss
- Instrument not calibrated or improperly calibrated
- Instrument not zeroed

Interpretation

- Unreasonable assumptions based upon unreasonable expectations (see text)
- Failure to establish accuracy required and achievable
- Patient-based examination stress (the "white coat hypertension")
- Hurried observation
- Observer bias
- Parallax
- "Smoothing" when recording

---

routine to check or set zero before initiating a measurement or a series of measurements.

Although this may seem obvious in relation to aneroid gauges, it is not perhaps immediately obvious to the user that a damaged sphygmomanometer may have lost some of its mercury and that the zero may be correspondingly offset.

Oscillometric/oscillotonometric approaches

Certain errors are relatively common in oscillometry and oscillotonometry. The first appearance of significant pointer deflection denotes the systolic point. The large pointer excursion which quickly follows the earlier deflection denotes the greater opening of the artery at a lower occlusion pressure. It is important to define properly the level at which the declining oscillation of the pointer represents the diastolic pressure. Letting the cuff pressure fall too rapidly, especially when the oscillations are reassuringly large, is a potent source of error in the diastolic reading. Necessary precautions include checking for leaks, especially in the tubing close to the connection points, and setting zero correctly before use.

> ### Common sources of error in oscillotonometry
>
> - Waiting for a large deflection before noting the systolic pressure
> - Failing to establish the proper indication of the diastolic level
> - Too rapid deflation of the cuff (do not open the valve too widely)
> - Failure to check for leaks (examine tubing and connections)
> - Failure to zero (always do it before use)

Plethysmography

Principles of application

The method in practice usually employs light sensing for detection, with the advantage that the sensor may be attached, provided due care is exercised; the sensing site otherwise demands no special attention, a boon when the site is relatively inaccessible.

The Finapres device

This device, described more fully in Chapter 7, has been adopted quite widely but, despite ease of attachment and convenience generally, it appears not to be without problems. It has been shown that it performs well only if the finger remains well perfused and it can be difficult to detect partial dislocation of the sensor. Moreover, correlation between actual pressures (as determined by direct means) and those obtained by the use of this method is inconsistent. However, it seems reasonable to conclude that the instrument is a competent follower of pressure trends, although not of the absolute values and, whilst subject to the usual problems associated with most indirect methods of blood pressure measurement, it is at its best when the subject is vasodilated.

Rigorous demands are placed on the cuff inflation controller, as it is required to change the cuff inflation pressure very rapidly indeed to every change in the plethysmograph signal. Not surprisingly, although the device works well under ideal conditions, it has often been found wanting under the more exacting circumstances prevailing in many real clinical situations.

115

Ultrasonic methods

Interface problems

Ultrasound is widely employed in medical practice, often under tightly controlled operating and environmental conditions.

The applications under review here rarely benefit from such ideal operating conditions, so that a number of considerations must be kept constantly in mind when blood pressure measuring equipment incorporating ultrasound is used.

The medium

Ultrasound requires a suitable medium. First, it is conducted poorly in air and is easily dissipated. Second, during passage from one medium to another, refraction of the ultrasound beam may take place. As the applications using ultrasound which concern us here often rely on the correct estimation of the angle of reflection of the ultrasound beam, this would be a major source of error. Suitable gels are used at the interface between ultrasound probe and skin to minimise both of these problems. Most suppliers furnish a proprietary gel or recommend a suitable interface material.

Contact

For the reasons just mentioned and, simply, to maintain continuity of the difficult interface, contact must be maintained at all times during a measurement or monitoring. The application of gels and other suitable media goes a long way towards this, but it is also necessary to ensure that contact is physically maintained by appropriate fixing.

Baseline setting

As with all forms of monitoring measurement, the measurement of blood pressure must be conducted against assurance that the baseline is zero. One of the intrinsic merits of the mercury sphygmomanometer is that the pool of mercury is self-levelling for practical purposes (provided none has been lost as a result of damage – which may be unnoticed). Inferential methods and methods which make only intermittent or occasional reference to atmospheric pressure, often only on specific intervention by the operator, are inherently liable to error due to lack of stable zero reference. Thus,

116

aneroid sphygmomanometers, oscillotonometers and oscillometers and all detectors intermittently obtaining indirect access to zero pressure reference, are susceptible. Similarly, electronic sensors calibrated against electrical reference variables, whilst often stable in use between routine calibrations, may occasionally drift during use. The moral is that, unless zero is established automatically (devices of this kind may produce error messages if zero calibration is unsatisfactory), users should make it a point of their routine practice to check zero before embarking on measurements or monitoring. The problem with blood pressure measuring instruments in this respect is that users too often regard them as "part of the furniture" and accord them less technical respect than, say, capnometers or the more glamorous intravascular measuring systems.

Electrical interference

Modern instruments for the monitoring of blood pressure are generally designed with the possibility of electrical interference much in mind. Nevertheless, some simple, stand-alone instruments may be designed for compactness and low price and be less satisfactory in this respect.

Interference may take several forms:

Mains interference

The mains supply has an alternating current frequency of 50 Hz. Poor design may permit this to be transmitted to the measuring or control system. More commonly, insufficient shielding permits transference of the effects of the field created by mains cables and mains-operated equipment to monitoring devices. The effects of this on blood pressure measuring devices is usually small, but the effects on electronic displays (for example, VDUs) of the values obtained and derived may be more severe and should be borne in mind in such circumstances. In these circumstances, displays may appear to quiver or "swim".

Electrostatic interference

Properly earthed equipment complying with the pertinent general standard requirements for electrical safety,[41] should pose no problems in respect of accumulated electric charge; this may be due to friction of certain materials in garments or to static discharge. However, equipment which is not earthed, yet properly complies with these same standards, for example double-insulated and "floating" equipment (isolated from the mains supply), may be the source of electrostatic discharge sufficient to affect displays in the manner described above.

Electromagnetic interference

Electromagnetic interference is produced by alternating current flowing along a conductor in proximity to a susceptible conductor or item of apparatus. Thus, unshielded mains cables and other electrical equipment, especially motorised equipment, may emit changing electromagnetic fields such as to induce stray signals into nearby measuring and monitoring equipment and their associated displays.[42,43]

Portable telephones, other types of radiotransmitters (for example, in ambulances and in fire and police vehicles), and certain types of computing and related equipment are potent sources of electromagnetic disturbance. In particular, microprocessor-based control and computation units and associated electronic displays may be seriously affected. Safe levels of this form of electromagnetic radiation are not yet established. However, a figure of 10 V per metre field strength has been widely canvassed. Portable telephones, for example, commonly emit more than 10 Vm^{-1}. They should therefore be switched off if carried in the vicinity of susceptible apparatus in operating theatre suites, recovery areas, critical care areas, clinics and ward areas, and elsewhere where important medical investigations are carried out.[44]

Defibrillation may be used on subjects who are undergoing monitoring, including blood pressure monitoring. In addition to the effects of the electrical current injected into the body at the time of defibrillation, there is considerable movement artefact in continuous blood pressure readings. However, these are relatively short-lived and other methods than blood pressure monitoring will take precedence in determining the adequacy of perfusion clinically.

1 Roche V, O'Malley K, O'Brien E. How "scientific" is blood pressure measurement in leading scientific journals? *J Hypertens* 1990: **8**: 1167–8.
2 Alpert S. Physiologic monitoring devices. *Crit Care Med* 1995; **23**: 1626–7.
3 Less JR, Alpert S, Nightingale SL. Institutional Review Boards and medical devices. *JAMA* 1994; **272**: 968–9.
4 Bruce NG, Shaper AG, Walker M, Wannamethee G. Observer bias in blood pressure studies. *J Hypertens* 1988; **6**: 375–80.
5 Curb JD, Labarthe DR, Cooper S, Cutter GR, Hawkins CM. Training and certification of observers. *Hypertension* 1983; **5**: 610–14.
6 O'Brien E, Mee F, Tan KS, Atkins N, O'Malley K. Training and assessment of observers for blood pressure measurement. *J Hum Hypertens* 1991; **5**: 7–10.
7 Rose G. Standardisation of observers in blood pressure measurement. *Lancet* 1965; **i**: 673–4.
8 Bland JM, Altman DG. Statistical methods for assessing agreement between two methods of clinical measurement. *Lancet* 1986; **1**: 307–10.

9 Barker WF, Hediger ML, Katz SH, Bowers EJ. Concurrent validity studies of blood pressure instrumentation: the Philadelphia Blood Pressure Project. *Hypertension* 1984; **6**: 85–91.

10 Garrow JS. Zero-muddler for unprejudiced sphygmomanometry. *Lancet* 1963; **iv**: 1205.

11 Fitzgerald D, O'Callaghan W, O'Malley K, O'Brien E. Inaccuracy in the London School of Hygeine Sphygmomanometer. *BMJ* 1982; **284**: 18–19.

12 De Gaudemaris R, Folsom AR, Prineas RJ, Luepker RV. The random zero versus the standard mercury sphygmomanometer: a systematic blood pressure difference. *Am J Epidemiol* 1985; **121**: 282–90.

13 Conroy R, O'Brien E, O'Malley K, Atkins N. Measurement error of the Hawksley Random zero sphygmomanometer: what damage has been done and what can we learn? *BMJ* 1993; **306**: 1319–22.

14 Conroy R, Atkins N, Mee F, O'Brien E, O'Malley K. Using Hawksley random zero sphygmomanometer as a gold standard may result in misleading conclusion. *Blood Pressure* 1994; **3**: 283–6.

15 Kinirons MT, Maskrey VL, Lawson M, Swift CG, Jackson SH. Hawksley random zero sphygmomanometer versus the standard sphygmomanometer: an investigation of the mechanisms. *J Hum Hypertens* 1995; **9**: 571–3.

16 Wright BM, Dore CF. A random zero sphygmomanometer. *Lancet* 1970; **1**: 337–8.

17 O'Brien E, Mee F, Atkins N, O'Malley K. Inaccuracy of the Hawksley Random Zero Sphygmomanometer. *Lancet* 1990; **336**: 1465–8.

18 Coalition for Critical Care Excellence. Consensus Conference on Physiologic Monitoring Devices: Standards of evidence for the safety and effectiveness of critical care monitoring devices and related interventions. *Crit Care Med* 1995; **23**: 1756–63.

19 O'Brien E, O'Malley K. Techniques for measuring blood pressure and their interpretation. In: Birkenhager W, ed. *Practical management of hypertension*. Dordrecht: Kluwer Academic Publishers, 1990.

20 Padfield PL, Jyothinagaram SG, Watson DM, Donald P, McGinley IM. Problems in the measurement of blood pressure. *J Hum Hypertens* 1990; **4** (Suppl. 2): 3–7.

21 Petrie J, Jamieson M, O'Brien E, Littler W, Padfield P, de Swiet M (for the Working Party on Blood Pressure Measurement). Videotape: *Blood pressure measurement*. London: BMJ Publishing Group, 1990.

22 O'Brien E, O'Malley K. Clinical blood pressure measurement. In: Birkenhager WH, Reid JL, series eds. *Handbook of hypertension*. Vol. 15. Robertson JIS, ed. *Clinical hypertension. Blood pressure measurement*. Amsterdam: Elsevier, 1992.

23 O'Brien E. Blood pressure measurement. In: Swales JD, ed. *Textbook of hypertension*. Oxford: Oxford Scientific Publications, 1994.

24 Rose GA. A sphygmomanometer for epidemiologists. *Lancet* 1964; **i**: 296–300.

25 Mancia G, Prati G, Pomidossi G *et al.* Doctor-ellicited blood pressure rises at the time of sphygmomanometric blood pressure assessment persist over repeated visits. *J Hypertens* 1985; **3** (Suppl. 3): S421–3.

26 Pickering TG, James GD, Boddie C, Harshfield GA, Blank S, Laragh, JH. How common is white coat hypertension? *JAMA* 1988; **2**: 584–6.

27 Gosse P, Promax H, Durandet P, Clementy J. "White coat" hypertension. No harm for the heart. *Hypertension* 1993; **22**: 766–70.

28 Middeke M, Schrader J. Nocturnal blood pressure in normotensive subjects and those with white coat, primary and secondary hypertension. *BMJ* 1994; **308**: 630–2.

29 de Swiet M, Dillon MJ, Littler W, O'Brien E, Padfield P, Petrie JC. Measurement of blood pressure in children. Recommendations of a Working Party of the British Hypertension Society. *BMJ* 1989; **299**: 497.

30 Sloan PJM, Zezulka A, Davies P, Sangal A, Beevers M, Beevers G. Standardised methods for comparison of sphygmomanometers. *J Hypertens* 1984; **2**: 547–51.

31 O'Brien E, Petrie J, Littler W *et al.* The British Hypertension Society protocol for the evaluation of automated and semi-automated blood pressure measuring devices with special reference to ambulatory systems. *J Hypertens* 1990; **8**: 607–19.

32 Ng KG, Small CF. Review of methods & simulators for evaluation of noninvasive blood pressure monitors. *J Clin Eng* 1992; **17**: 469–79. (Errata appear in *J Clin Eng* 1993; **18**: 37 and 1994; **19**: 132.)

119

33 O'Brien E, Atkins N, Mee F, O'Malley K. Evaluation of blood pressure measuring devices. *Clin Exp Hypertens* 1993; **15**: 1087–97.

34 O'Brien E, Petrie J, Littler WA *et al*. An outline of the British Hypertension Society Protocol for the evaluation of blood pressure measuring devices. *J Hypertens* 1993; **11**: 677–9.

35 O'Brien E, Petrie J, Littler WA *et al*. Protocol for the evaluation of blood pressure measuring devices. *J Hypertens* 1993; **11** (Suppl. 1); S43–63.

36 Reid J. Validation of blood pressure measuring systems. *J Hypertens* 1993; **11**: 1–11.

37 Iyriboz Y, Hearon CM. A proposal for scientific validation of instruments for indirect blood pressure measurement at rest, during exercise, and in critical care. *J Clin Monit* 1994; **10**: 163–77.

38 Ng KG, Small CF. Update on methods & simulators for evaluation of noninvasive blood pressure monitors. *J Clin Eng* 1994; **19**: 125–34.

39 O'Brien E, O'Malley K, Atkins N, Mee F. A review of validation procedures for blood pressure measuring devices. In: Waeber B, O'Brien E, O'Malley K, Brunner HR, eds. *Ambulatory blood pressure*. New York: Raven Press, 1994.

40 O'Brien E, Atkins N. A comparison of the BHS and AAMI protocols for validating blood pressure measuring devices: can the two be reconciled? *J Hypertens* 1994; **12**: 1089–94.

41 IEC 601-1 (EN60601-1, BS 5724, Pt. 1). *Medical electrical equipment. Part I: General requirements for safety*. Geneva: International Electrotechnical Commission, 1988.

42 IEC 1000-4-2 (BS EN 61000-4-2). *Section 2: Electrostatic discharges. Immunity test*. Geneva: International Electrotechnical Commission, 1997.

43 IEC 1000-4-3 (BS EN 61000-4-3). *Section 3: Immunity to radiated RF electrical fields*. Geneva: International Electrotechnical Commission, 1997.

44 Safety Action Bulletin: SAB(94)49. *Portable cordless and cellular telephones: interference with medical devices*. London: Department of Health, November 1994.

9 Diagnostic scope and limitations of blood pressure monitoring

Medical

Hospital

All the techniques described may be used in the hospital setting. Most familiar is the Riva-Rocci method, using either a mercury or an aneroid manometer. When in the hands of trained diligent users, the method is reliable and repeatable for the purposes of clinical interpretation and subsequent action. The errors have been described in Chapter 8, but the weaknesses of the method in practice lie in the often poor condition of the equipment, such as leaks in the tubing, valve and elsewhere, and failure to ensure a true zero reference. Delegation to inexperienced or even untrained users must place recordings thus obtained in doubt. Routine charting must not be synonymous with lax measurement.

Automated measurements are most often undertaken in areas in which repeated measurements need to be made. The advantages of hard-copy output, when this is available with the apparatus, are evident. Provided the apparatus is well maintained and properly applied to the subject, the results may be expected to be clinically satisfactory. Precautions should be taken to protect the patient from potential injury resulting from repeated cuff inflation (see Chapters 5 and 6).

Adults

In addition to the foregoing considerations, adults may be apprehensive about the results of blood pressure measurements and their therapeutic and social implications. A relaxed and reassuring approach to the subject is essential in such circumstances. This, in any case, should be a normal accompaniment to blood pressure measurement, as it may be impossible to determine at a glance which subjects are apprehensive for serious underlying reasons as distinct from transient anxiety traceable to simply having just arrived at the hospital or being confronted by a white coat.[1,2]

Paediatrics

Especial care is necessary when obtaining estimations of blood pressure in children. There is continuing argument about the threat or otherwise seen by children in doctors and others in white coats, nurses in uniform and the like. It should be appreciated also that children have different reasons for apprehension from those of adults. Of special note is the embarrassment felt by older children, say between 8 and 13 years, when in an environment where they feel very insecure compared to the certainty they feel in familiar environments such as the school and home. A matter-of-fact, genuinely interested approach is often well rewarded and the subject should be made aware that the tightness of the inflated cuff is quite normal.

Small children and infants may have "podgy" limbs. It is important to identify the position of the artery accurately, so far as is possible, and to ensure that the cuff is of the correct size. Movement due to restlessness may be a problem and gentle conversation, whether or not properly understood by the smallest subjects, may be sufficient to gain their attention and, hence, effective cooperation. The presence of a parent or other trusted person is often advantageous.

The special problems encountered when making blood pressure measurements in neonates, infants, and small children, combined with their chubbiness and the lower pressures obtaining in these groups, when compared with those in adults, make for difficulties in establishing whether or not readings may be valid. For this reason, the flush method (see Chapter 4) has attained a degree of popularity. Again, however, some of the newer automated devices are better adapted to these problems of measurement than formerly.

Emergencies

In the face of extreme urgency and when only the most basic equipment is available, the simple expedient of obtaining a crude estimate of the systolic blood pressure by arterial occlusion and *palpation* of a peripheral pulse should not be overlooked. Whilst it is true that the systolic pressure is not a good indicator of the adequacy of perfusion, the systolic value obtained when combined with the quality of the pulse may give useful instant information. All that is required is a sphygmomanometer cuff and manometer. The aneroid device is especially convenient in these circumstances. The measurement may then proceed to formal *auscultation*, provided the subject is accessible and reasonably still – conditions not universal in emergency settings. Where aneroid manometers are carried by

122

emergency teams, it is essential that they be subjected to routine *calibration checks*.

Automated blood pressure measurement equipment is increasingly available for use in emergencies. When used correctly and under acceptable conditions, it undoubtedly has a place. At the same time, the limitations imposed by shock states, arrhythmias, movement artefact, and the other sources of error referred to earlier (see Chapter 8) must be borne in mind. When several users are involved in a given emergency, it must be ensured that displayed values are indeed recently updated values and not those retained from an earlier measurement cycle. The improvements which have been made in artefact rejection and the ruggedness and reliability of many current designs is likely to promote their popularity in emergency applications. In particular, small, lightweight, *hand-held* devices have attractions.

Under emergency conditions of shock, trauma, and sudden critical illness, cardiac output may be severely reduced, blood volume may be depleted, and vasoconstriction is often present. All the non-invasive methods of determining the blood pressure are handicapped in such circumstances, as all depend to a greater or lesser extent on changes in the calibre of the arteries and a pulsatile flow (the greater the pulse pressure the better). In the elderly and in subjects with hypertensive and other arteriopathies, the distensibility of the vessels may also be reduced. In critical illness with these features, non-invasive monitoring is no substitute for intra-arterial monitoring.

Therefore, the limitations of indirect methods of blood pressure measurement when the perfusion is poor, cardiac output reduced, or the patient vasoconstricted must be kept in mind constantly. At the same time, sequential measurements under the same conditions may be expected to reveal trends and approximate ranges, whether manual or automated methods are employed. Access may be restricted and measurements from cuffs applied over clothing may be misleading. Although speed may be necessary, invalid readings resulting in incorrect responses are no substitute for exercising a little more care and effort to obtain valid readings. In the event that access to a convenient large artery is impracticable, the value of palpation of the radial or dorsalis pedis pulses, as a means of detecting perfusion at or near the systolic blood pressure level, should not be forgotten. Automatic monitoring is of value in certain situations, such as during rapid blood and colloid administration,[3] as in the initial treatment of burns,[4] and has been found satisfactory during the emergency transport of the critically ill,[5] including children.[6] Indeed, there seems to be no reason why automated blood pressure measuring instruments should not be used in circumstances where fall-back methods are available and the observers are highly skilled. As usual, note should be taken of the frequency of measurements, to avoid gratuitous injury to a limb. Means should be provided with permanently mounted (e.g. wall-mounted) instruments to enable them to be correctly positioned in relation to the patient.

Ambulances

Ambulance services may choose to standardise on particular types of blood pressure measuring apparatus. The apparatus should be thus chosen with reference to susceptibility to shock, impact, and vibration, and to whether or not it will be fixed or free-standing. It may be assumed that all personnel using or responsible for such equipment will be properly trained in its care and use.

Special applications

Critical care

In many critical care settings, provided there is a valid indication for indirect blood pressure measurement, the use of some automated instruments brings with it the provision of output signals which may be fed into a monitoring system or a dedicated recorder, in order that permanent records may be held and data processing may be undertaken. Care should be taken that the interface arrangements are appropriate and that the environment is suitable for the satisfactory transfer of the pertinent signals.

Coronary care

Whilst the detection of arrhythmias, including cardiac arrest is clearly of the greatest importance, the measurement of blood pressure will often be of secondary importance. Where the stability of blood pressure is uncertain or cardiac output is poor or fluctuating, indirect methods properly applied may be satisfactory, but the possible need for continuous direct arterial monitoring should be considered. Again, in this group, sleep disturbance is a potentially serious problem when measurements are needed frequently; thus a balance needs to be struck between regular information and damaging disturbance.

Intensive care

Whilst most measurements of blood pressure in the critically ill are likely to be made using direct cannulation of vessels associated with dedicated transducers, there is a place for indirect methods. Many patients have life-threatening conditions which do not directly affect the cardiovascular system; in these cases blood pressure measurement is undertaken largely to exclude cardiovascular involvement or deterioration. Disturbance of sleep in unsedated patients when measurements, including blood pressure measurements need to be made, is a significant problem in critical care. It is a moot point whether the gentle approach of a concerned nurse or doctor or the regular, relatively non-intrusive repetition of the automated device constitutes the better option. This is not a problem when direct invasive monitoring is being used.

Obstetrics/pregnancy

Automatic blood pressure monitoring is commonly used in pregnancy, especially in the event of pre-eclampsia, where the frequency of measurements must be limited in order to avoid undue interruption of the perfusion of the limb bearing the cuff,[7] and during delivery under epidural analgesia. Monitoring may also be of value outside the delivery suite.[8]

Ambulatory monitoring

Ambulatory monitoring has grown in popularity in recent years to the extent that it deserves to be dealt with separately. Moreover, it is not confined to hospital or general practice, but is used wherever sufficient enthusiasm and understanding exists on the part of staff and patients. It forms the content of Chapter 10.

General practice

Given that measurements of blood pressure in general practice are made principally for the purposes of diagnosis, screening,[9] and follow-up, it is important to achieve high accuracy whenever possible.[10] Whilst trends are important, it is the long-term impact of such trends that matters, rather than the minute to minute changes seen in some forms of acute illness. Thus, individual readings may be widely spaced in time and considerable reliance placed on them in terms of instituting or modifying therapy. Time spent in ensuring that the measurements are accurate is time well spent.[11]

Public health aspects

General practice is well placed to assist in screening of patients in the practice, for example for hypertension.[9,12] Wider surveys may, of course, be mounted as part of the epidemiological study of communities in public health programmes.[13-16] Alternatively, studies may be part of clinical audit or critical incident monitoring surveys.[17]

Practical choices

The possible benefits of automated devices in the doctor's surgery and, perhaps more especially, of portable hand-held instruments in the home, should be borne in mind. However, the traditional Riva-Rocci method is still justly popular. It may be argued that the interaction necessary between doctor or practice nurse and patient provides the best conditions for a careful measurement to be carried out. Note should be taken of the variations in pressure which take place during normal breathing when decisions are made as to what accuracy to read the scale. Excellent guidance on this and related matters is given in the *ABC of Hypertension*.[18]

Precautions in use

Mercury sphygmomanometers should be checked frequently for air leaks, and measurements should not be accepted in the presence of proven or suspected leaks. Similarly, aneroid sphygmomanometers should be routinely checked for leaks and, in addition, they should be examined for external damage, where the effects may not be immediately apparent, and calibrated against standards from time to time. Automated instruments, especially easily damaged portable devices, should be checked and calibrated according to the manufacturer's or supplier's instructions.

Nursing

Institutional

The measurement of blood pressure is routine in wards and departments. To the extent that it is routine, it is prone to being regarded as perfunctory and is likely to be delegated. Thus, it is probable that a measurement believed to be of great importance may be undertaken without a clear knowledge of its principles and practice. Moreover, the meticulousness surrounding the measurement when undertaken by a specialist physician dealing with hypertension may contrast markedly with the casual manner in which subsequent follow-up estimations may be made. Perhaps this is most evident when routine sphygmomanometry is undertaken. It is common experience that the ward or department sphygmomanometer may be old, ill-used and even overtly damaged. Yet, it "belongs" to no-one and may be regarded as satisfactory if it seems to work at all. Features commonly noted include containers which fail to protect the contents properly and leaks in the bulb or tubing such as to render controlled deflation difficult or impossible. Failure to observe reasonable rules of use sometimes results in breakage of the glass tube containing the mercury column with consequent escape of the highly toxic contents. All concerned should ensure that equipment is up to standard and that all staff who use sphygmomanometers are trained in their correct use and are aware of the possible errors and their implications.

Although oscillometers and oscillotonometers are precision instruments, they are not always handled with due care. Damage may affect the delicate transmission apparatus between aneroid and display needle or may render the occlusion/deflating valve faulty. They should not be used as a substitute for a tourniquet, for which purpose they are neither designed nor suitable.

The newer automated devices are generally built to a good standard and by virtue of their shape, size, and construction are generally less susceptible to misuse than the portable instruments. Being electrical and more advanced than the basic instrumentation, they perhaps command rather more respect from users also. In this case, however, the hazards devolve more upon lack of familiarity with any operational foibles which they may have. In particular, the fact that they conveniently display numerical values may confer upon them, in the eyes of inexperienced users, a blind faith in the accuracy of the data presented. It needs to be stressed that such machines should be subject to routine maintenance and calibration checks, and that users should be trained to correlate the output with reasonable expectations, so that they do not believe and act upon the displayed values indiscriminately. Further, the algorithms which underlie the operation of these devices necessarily must make provision for failed and dubious estimations, owing to subject movement or other artefact. In some instances also, instruments retain the display from a previous reading if not reset and may then instill unwarranted confidence when use is continuous, as in the operating theatre, recovery area, or the cardiac monitoring setting. Some miniaturised versions of automated blood pressure recording apparatus have appeared from time to time. Some have been shown to be better than others, but the best are comparable with their larger counterparts.[19]

It is important to note that there is now a European Standard,[20] with which all indirect blood pressure measuring equipment should comply when first purchased. Other standards are also available.[21-27] It is incumbent on purchasers to ensure that they are aware of the range of equipment available and its suitability for the intended application, that proper procedures are invoked for its acquisition and commissioning, that users are trained in its correct use and are updated as necessary, and that the equipment is properly and regularly maintained.[28,29]

Community

Many of the considerations noted above apply to the community. Whilst sphygmomanometers have been the mainstay in the past, it seems likely that the small, lightweight automated apparatus now available will appear in the community in greater numbers in primary care and in the community at large. The attraction to general practitioners and community nurses is apparent.

Problems of the "nurse on-the-move"

The busy community nurse encounters conditions which are different from those obtaining in institutions and general practitioners' surgeries. They are frequently more demanding, in that the nurse may be engaged in active practical procedures in the care of patients and may be constantly on the move for much of the working day. Given that more responsibility than ever is devolving upon community nurses, as hospitals endeavour to discharge patients earlier than previously, and more of the duties once regarded as the province of doctors, such as following up patients with specific conditions like hypertension, are being performed by community nurses, the equipment they use and the training they receive in its use should be appropriate. Thus, small compact and rugged equipment should be the order of the day where practicable. Many community nurses are already very familiar with the benefits of communications and the use of computers, static and portable. Matching measuring equipment will be a great boon to them.

Hard copy and communications

Blood pressure measuring devices incorporating miniature printers have a special attraction in providing a permanent record, whilst devices with a communications interface (for example, RS-232) are ideal for the collecting and subsequent uploading of data[30] to a portable computer or to a central office, or departmental computer for subsequent analysis and inclusion in patients' records.

Practical solutions

Several portable devices are already available, but not all have hard-copy output and few have communications facilities. Although such models may have crude instruction sheets, comprehensive manuals are not yet the norm. Better still, the trend for institutional monitoring instruments to have basic instructions for use printed on them or attached to them

128

should become the norm. Tough but flexible pull-out instruction "sheets", incorporated into the body of the device are especially useful.

Possible improvements

Besides the derived data that automated instruments often yield in the form of pulse rate, mean pressure, and the time of the measurement, the extrapolation of the so-called "area under the curve", representing the sequential digital values produced during measurement by instruments using constant cuff deflation, might be of value in the initial assessment of shocked and other hypotensive patients, and in the crude information it might yield about the condition of the peripheral vasculature in arteriopaths and hypertensives. As is so often the case, the technology is waiting to be exploited, but the limitations imposed are those of clinicians and others being unaware of what might be done or genuinely doubtful about the real usefulness of such additional data and parameters.

Other professional groups

"Spot"-checking

Blood pressure measurement is perhaps more dependent upon the competence and specifically informed state of the person making the measurement than on his or her status. As with other measurements and procedures usually undertaken only in hospital or in the doctor's office or surgery, there may be a case for the extension of the necessary skills to others, for example physiotherapists, who could perform this valuable measurement when the opportunity presented.

Screening

Similarly, screening programs have often involved highly trained paramedical personnel. Screening of the blood pressure of particular groups, "at-risk", or more general, has been undertaken and need not necessarily be conducted only by medical or nursing staff. The emergence of suitable apparatus may be an added incentive.

Role of paramedical personnel

Many patients who become ill suddenly are attended by emergency paramedical ambulance crews. Such trained personnel now routinely set up drips and pass tracheal tubes. Among their equipment, automated blood pressure apparatus, along with suitable training in its use, would be a valuable asset.

Possible role of pharmacists

Increasingly, pharmacists (especially in hospital) are undertaking roles in relation to the supervision of patients whose drug treatment they dispense. It remains to be seen whether those receiving therapy for hypertension and related cardiovascular disorders might have their blood pressure surveillance carried out by such a group.[31]

Hygiene

Blood pressure cuffs may harbour bacteria and the possibility of transmission of infection should be kept in mind.[32]

1 Mancia G, Prati G, Pomidossi G *et al.* Doctor-elicited blood pressure rises at the time of sphygmomanometric blood pressure assessment persist over repeated visits. *J Hypertens* 1985; **3** (Suppl. 3): S421–3.
2 Pickering TG, James GD, Boddie C, Harshfield GA, Blank S, Laragh, JH. How common is white coat hypertension? *JAMA* 1988; **2**: 584–6.
3 Cusack S, Moulton C, Swann IJ. The introduction of automatic blood pressure monitoring to an accident and emergency resuscitation room. *Arch Emerg Med* 1993; **10**: 39–42.
4 Bainbridge LC, Simmons HM, Elliot D. The use of automatic blood pressure monitors in the burned patient. *Brit J Plast Surg* 1990; **43**: 322–4.
5 Runcie CJ, Reeve W, Reidy J, Dougall JR. A comparison of measurements of blood pressure, heart-rate and oxygenation during inter-hospital transport of the critically ill. *Intens Care Med* 1990; **16**: 317–22.
6 Barry PW, Ralston C. Adverse events occurring during interhospital transfer of the critically ill. *Arch Dis Child* 1994; **71**: 8–11.
7 Quinn M. Automated blood pressure measurement devices: a potential source of morbidity in preeclampsia? *Amer J Obstet Gynecol* 1994; **170**: 1303–7.
8 Smith CV, Selig CL, Rayburn WF, Yi PF. Reliability of compact electronic blood pressure monitors for hypertensive pregnant women. *J Reprod Med* 1990; **35**: 399–401.
9 Barber JH, Beevers DG, Fife R, Hawthorne VM, McKenzie HM, Sinclair RG. Blood pressure screening and supervision in general practice. *BMJ* 1979; **i**: 843–6.
10 Burke MJ, Towers H, O'Malley K, Fitzgerald DJ, O'Brien RT. Sphygmomanometers in hospital and family practice: problems and recommendations. *BMJ* 1982; **285**: 469–71.
11 Beevers DG, Marshall HJ. In: O'Brien ET, Beevers DG, Marshall HJ, eds. *ABC of Hypertension*, 3rd edn. London: BMJ Publishing Group, 1995: 69.
12 Staessen J, Fagard R, Amery A. Body weight and blood pressure. *J Human Hypertens* 1989; **2**: 209–18.
13 Hart JT. *Hypertension: community control of high blood pressure*, 3rd edn. Oxford: Radcliffe Medical Press, 1993.
14 Hawthorne VM, Greaves DA, Beevers DG. Blood pressure in a Scottish town. *BMJ* 1974; **3**: 600–3.
15 Rose G. Strategy of prevention: lessons from cardiovascular disease. *BMJ* 1981; **282**: 1847–51. (Commented on by: Swales JD. Primary care at the centre. *J Roy Soc Med* 1995; **88**: 425.)

16 Whelton PK, Klag MJ. Blood pressure in Westernized populations. In: Swales JD, ed. *Textbook of hypertension*. Oxford: Blackwell Scientific Publications, 1994: 14.

17 Cockings JGL, Webb RK, Klepper ID, Currie M, Morgan C. Blood pressure monitoring – applications and limitations: an analysis of 2,000 incident reports. *Anaesth Intens Care* 1993; **21**: 565–9.

18 O'Brien ET, Beevers, DG, Marshall HJ, eds. *ABC of Hypertension* 3rd ed. London: BMJ Publishing Group, 1995.

19 Johnson CJM, Kerr JM. Automatic blood pressure monitors. A clinical evaluation of five models in adults. *Anaesthesia* 1985; **40**: 471–8.

20 CEN standard EN 1060 Non-invasive sphygmomanometers: EN 1060–1 Part 1: General requirements; EN 1060–2 Part 2: Supplementary requirements for mechanical sphygmomanometers; EN 1060–3 Part 3: Supplementary requirements for electromechanical blood pressure measuring systems. Brussels: Committée Européen de Normalisation (CEN) (in preparation).

21 Federal specifications for sphygmomanometers: aneroid and mercurial. Washington DC: Superintendent of Documents, 1978. US Government Printing Office GG-S-618D.

22 American National Standard for Non-automated sphygmomanometers. Arlington, Va: Association for the Advancement of Medical Instrumentation (under revision). (Commentary appears in Prisant LM, Alpert BS, Robbins CB, *et al.* American National Standard for nonautomated sphygmomanometers. Summary report. *Amer J Hypertens* 1995; **8**: 210–13.)

23 American National Standard for Electronic or automated sphygmomanometers. ANSI/AAMI SP 10–1992. Arlington, Va: Association for the Advancement of Medical Instrumentation, 1993. (Commentary appears in White WB, Berson AS, Robbins C *et al.* National standard for measurement of resting and ambulatory blood pressure with automated sphygmomanometers. *Hypertension* 1993; **21**: 504–9.)

24 Australian Standard: Sphygmomanometers (No. AS 3655–1989): 36. North Sydney: Australian Standards Association, 1989.

25 British Standards Institution. Specification for aneroid and mercury non-automated sphygmomanometers (Revision of BS 2743 and BS 2744). London: British Standards Institution, 1990. (Superseded by CEN standards, *q.v.*)

26 IEC 601–2–30. Particular requirements for the safety of automatic cycling indirect blood pressure monitoring equipment. Geneva: International Electrotechnical Commission, 1995.

27 IEC 930. Guidance for administrative, medical, and nursing staff concerned with the safe use of medical electrical equipment. Geneva: International Electrotechnical Commission, 1988.

28 The report of the Expert Working Group on alarms on clinical monitors. London, Medical Devices Agency, 1995: 11–23.

29 Medical Devices Directorate. Health Equipment Information No. 98. Management of medical equipment and devices. London: Department of Health, 1991.

30 Nickalls RWD, Ramasubramanian R. Interfacing the IBM-PC to medical equipment. The art of serial communication. Cambridge: Cambridge University Press, 1995.

31 Nykamp D, Barnett CW. Use of stationary automated blood pressure devices in pharmacies. *Amer Pharm* 1992; **NS32**(6): 33–6.

32 Arnold WP Hug CC. Recommendations for infection control for the practice of anesthesiology. Park Ridge, Illinois: American Society of Anesthesiologists, 1991.

10 Ambulatory non-invasive blood pressure monitoring

Note: Ambulatory monitoring is a relatively new way of measuring blood pressure and the literature is extensive but diffuse, reflecting a wide divergence of opinion. In this chapter, only a representative selection of studies is referenced.

There has been interest since the 1970s in the possibility of monitoring patients' blood pressures outside the hospital, as they go about their normal activities. Where this was under the supervision of the patient's physician, there were obvious benefits to be obtained by continuous blood pressure monitoring. Although the early approaches required direct arterial cannulation, with the attendant problems of maintaining flushing systems and ensuring correct calibration, more recent methods of measurement have opened up the possibility of making devices both non-invasive and portable, to the point where they are now miniaturised and may be kept conveniently on the person. The advantages were set out by Parati *et al.*[1] How patients respond to therapy when they return home from hospital or from the out-patient clinic,[2] and whether specific activities or varieties of stress affect their responses can now be determined.[3] In particular, in the light of early experience, it became feasible to examine the 24-hour ambulatory blood pressure records of patients, including diurnal variations,[4-6] and to investigate the behaviour of the blood pressure in specific medical conditions, such as diabetes, pregnancy, and hypertension, as well as in the elderly and in the setting of general practice. As a result, the technique has been applied to a variety of situations in which it is convenient to measure and/or record the blood pressure repeatedly or continuously without the need for the patient to attend a clinic for that purpose alone.

The ambulatory monitoring of response to treatment of hypertension

Coats *et al.* gave an account of experience with the ambulatory monitoring of patients' responses to antihypertensive drugs.[7] Since then, there have been many similar accounts demonstrating the benefits of the approach.

132

Subsequent decision-making in relation to drug therapy has been influenced by the data gathered.[8,9]

Giles looked ahead to the possibilities of linking this kind of monitoring to clinical trials.[10] Indeed, Conway had already commented on the usefulness of ambulatory blood pressure monitoring both in therapy and associated clinical trials.[11] One of the problems of drug trials, the need for a placebo, was discussed by Raftery,[12] who observed that, whereas a trial making a comparison with direct measurement might not require it, a placebo was necessary when indirect measurements, such as ambulatory monitoring, were used. Some authorities have recommended that ambulatory monitoring should in any case be used in trials of antihypertensive drugs.[13,14]

Paediatric ambulatory monitoring

This has been described in general terms;[15] in respect of 24-hour ambulatory monitoring;[16,17] in the detection of borderline hypertension;[18] in sleep apnoea;[19] and after renal transplantation.[20]

Use in the elderly

There are particular attractions in ambulatory monitoring in the elderly, for example, the ambulatory detection of myocardial ischaemia[21] and the monitoring of the relationship between hypertension and obesity in the elderly.[22]

Miscellaneous conditions

Ambulatory blood pressure monitoring has been reported in the monitoring of phaeochromocytoma,[23] and has been used in surveillance of stressful occupations,[24] where it was possible to show that telephone operators displayed less stress-related hypertension during periods of heavy workload than when waiting for calls.[25]

Are ambulatory records as good as clinic measurements?

Following a multi-centre study,[26] there have been reports indicating that the data obtained by ambulatory blood pressure monitoring are as good as or superior to those obtained in the doctor's office or surgery.[27-29] Between visits, variability was found to be similar using ambulatory or casual reading methods.[30] It is believed that the absence of the "white coat" syndrome from the picture may contribute substantially to the apparent success of ambulatory monitoring, but the evidence is inconclusive.[31,32]

Prediction of target-organ disease or injury

The assessment of patients deemed to be at risk of complications from hypertension is difficult when based upon isolated readings taken in the clinic. Ambulatory monitoring may be thought to have advantages in this connection and, certainly, ambulatory monitoring complements casual readings. Some authors have commented on the efficacy of ambulatory monitoring in high-risk hypertensives,[9,33,34] but others have noted that, whilst certain groups may benefit specifically, it is imprudent to generalise.[35] The approach has been applied to the prediction of hypertension. However, a nationwide US study observed that while ambulatory monitoring was valuable in the prediction of end-organ damage, it was not cost-effective in the monitoring of newly diagnosed hypertensives,[36] a finding tempered by the cost-effectiveness of the approach in the management of established hypertension.[29,37]

Validity of ambulatory blood pressure monitoring

A major concern is the validity of the data.[38] Criteria have been suggested for the manner in which data are obtained.[39] Moreover, there is uncertainty about what constitutes normal values, and several studies have been concerned with attempts to establish them.[40-49] One has shown that ambulatory indirect blood pressure monitoring yields less satisfactory results than direct intra-arterial ambulatory monitoring,[50] while another demonstrated no appreciable difference.[51] These findings must, however, be set against the difficulties of maintaining ambulatory direct monitoring. Pickering has urged that ambulatory monitoring is capable of reducing the errors associated with blood pressure measurement by conventional means when the methodology is satisfactory.[52] Problems in the methodology were addressed by Zurmann.[53] Errors may also be introduced by changes in posture during sleep and during the waking hours, with changes in activity, and as a result of environmental factors.[54] Concern that the disturbance to sleep occasioned by measurements may detract from their value has largely been dispelled.[55,56] When the data are recorded automatically, it is possible to identify all the relevant phases.[56] The period during which ambulatory monitoring takes place is of some importance. It has been shown that 24-hour monitoring is superior to monitoring over 1 hour only,[57] but that

134

4-hour periods are better;[58] 24-hour data have been validated against the 24-hour electrocardiogram in a study that showed good correlation between the ambulatory methods of recording and sphygmomanometry.[59]

Validation data have been produced[60] and methods of statistical analysis considered.[61] It has been pointed out that care must be exercised when "smoothing" of data is contemplated.[62] Further, a threat to validity may lie in subtle software changes insufficient to have prompted a change of model of the monitor offered for sale.[63]

It may be that ambulatory monitoring needs further validation.[64] Nevertheless, its cost-effectiveness in the management of hypertension has already been referred to and its overall cost-effectiveness as a clinical technique has also been confirmed.[65,66]

Clinical views on ambulatory blood pressure monitoring

This has been assessed,[67–71] and it was considered satisfactory in the practices of both the hospital[72] and primary care physician.[73] A nursing view has been expressed.[74] The feasibility of adapting the ambulatory monitoring technique to exercise testing has been explored, but with less than satisfactory results.[75] It should be noted that, although activity may have only a limited effect on the validity of the results, the presence of the device may restrict the individual's activity.[76] Complications reported include subjective sleep disturbance,[77] petechiae and ecchymoses,[78] and nerve damage.[79]

Design and evaluation of equipment

Hansen has queried whether the design of equipment intended for ambulatory blood pressure monitoring is adequate.[63] The subject has been too extensively reviewed for discussion in this book. Appendix A to this chapter provides full references and commentary on the studies so far published.[68,80–91]

A wide variety of equipment has appeared over the years. The majority of devices have been based on the oscillometric principle, while plethysmography and tonometry have also been used. Many have been reviewed. The references quoted in Appendix B to this chapter sometimes cover several devices and are in approximately chronological order.[92–165]

1 Parati G, Mutti E, Ravogli A, Trazzi S, Villani A, Mancia G. Advantages and disadvantages of non-invasive ambulatory blood pressure monitoring. *J Hypertens* 1990; **8** (Suppl): S33–8.

2 Waeber B, Scherrer U, Petrillo A *et al.* Are some hypertensives overtreated? A prospective study of ambulatory blood pressure recording. *Lancet* 1987; **ii**: 32–4.

3 Davies RJO, Jenkins N, Stradling JR. Effects of measuring ambulatory blood pressure on sleep and blood pressure during sleep. *BMJ* 1994; **308**: 820–3.

4 O'Brien E, Sheridan J, O'Malley K. Dippers and non-dippers. *Lancet* 1988; **ii**: 397.

5 Pickering TG. The clinical significance of diurnal pressure variations: dippers and non-dippers. *Circulation* 1990; **81**: 700–2.

6 Staessen J, Bulpitt CJ, O'Brien E *et al.* The diurnal blood pressure profile: a population study. *Am J Hypertens* 1992; **5**: 386–92.

7 Coats AJ, Conway J, Somers VK, Isea JE, Sleight P. Ambulatory pressure monitoring in the assessment of antihypertensive therapy. *Cardiovasc Drugs Ther* 1989; 3 (Suppl. 1): 303–11.

8 Whelton A. Application of ambulatory blood pressure monitoring to clinical therapeutic decisions in hypertension. *J Hypertens* 1991; **9** (Suppl.): S21–5.

9 Whelton A. Ambulatory blood pressure monitoring: a new window to decision-making in hypertension. *Clin Cardiol* 1992; **15** (Suppl. 2): II 14–17.

10 Giles TD. Future uses of ambulatory blood pressure monitoring: implications for therapy. *Clin Cardiol* 1992; **15** (Suppl. 2): II18–21.

11 Conway J, Coats A, Radaelli A. Ambulatory blood pressure in relation to drug treatment and clinical trials. *J Hypertens* 1990; **8** (Suppl.): S83–5.

12 Raftery EB, Gould BA. The effect of placebo on indirect and direct blood pressure measurements. *J Hypertens* 1990; **8** (Suppl.): S93–100.

13 Conway J, Coats AJ. Ambulatory blood pressure monitoring in the design of antihypertensive drug trials. *J Hypertens* 1991; **9** (Suppl.): S57–8.

14 Lipicky R. The United States Food and Drug Administration guidelines on ambulatory blood pressure monitoring. *J Hypertens* 1991; **9** (Suppl.): S59.

15 Harshfield GA, Alpert BS, Pulliam DA, Somes GW, Wilson DK. Ambulatory blood pressure recordings in children and adolescents. *Pediatrics* 1994; **94**: 180–4.

16 Krull F, Buck T, Offner G, Brodehl J. Twenty-four hour blood pressure monitoring in healthy children. *Eur J Pediatr* 1993; **152**: 555–8.

17 Nicholson WR, Matthews JN, O'Sullivan JJ, Wren C. Ambulatory blood pressure monitoring. *Arch Dis Child* 1993; **69**: 681–4.

18 Loirat C, Azancot-Benisty A, Bossu C, Durand I. Value of ambulatory blood pressure monitoring in borderline hypertension in the child. *Ann Pediatr (Paris)* 1991; **38**: 381–6.

19 Noda A, Okada T, Hayashi H, Yasuma F, Yokota M. 24-hour ambulatory blood pressure variability in obstructive sleep apnea syndrome. *Chest* 1993; **103**: 1343–7.

20 Soergel M, Maisin A, Azancot-Benisty A, Loirat C. Ambulatory blood pressure measurement in children and adolescents with kidney transplants. *Z Kardiol* 1992; **81** (Suppl 2.): 67–70.

21 Trenkwalder P, Dobrindt R, Plaschke M, Lydtin H. Usefulness of simultaneous ambulatory electrocardiographic and blood pressure monitoring in detecting myocardial ischemia in patients > 70 years of age with systemic hypertension. *Amer J Cardiol* 1993; **72**: 927–31.

22 Guagnano MT, Merlitti D, Murri R, Palitti VP, Sensi S. Ambulatory blood pressure monitoring in evaluating the relationship between obesity and blood pressure. *J Hum Hypertens* 1994; **8**: 245–50.

23 Katoh K. A study on blood pressure variation – the clinical validation of continuous direct blood pressure recording in patients with pheochromocytoma. *Hokkaido Igaku Zasshi* 1991; **66**: 769–79.

24 Blumenthal JA, Thyrum ET, Siegel WC. Contribution of job strain, job status and marital status to laboratory and ambulatory blood pressure in patients with mild hypertension. *J Psychosom Res* 1995; **39**: 133–44.

25 Nielsen HW. Continuous monitoring of pulse and blood pressure among telephone operators. *Ugeskr Laeger* 1994; **156**: 5866–9.

26 Clement DL. Office versus ambulatory recordings of blood pressure (OvA): a European multicenter study. The Steering Committee. *J Hypertens* 1990; **8** (Suppl.): S39–41.

27 Enstrom-Granath I. Ambulatory blood pressure monitoring. A tool for more comprehensive assessment. *Blood Press* 1992; **5** (Suppl.): 1–27.

28 Veerman DP, van Montfrans GA. Nurse-measured or ambulatory blood pressure in routine hypertension care. *J Hypertens* 1993; **11**: 287–92.

29 Bottini PB, Prisant LM, Carr AA. Automated blood pressure monitoring. Should it be used routinely in managing hypertension? *Postgrad Med* 1994; **95**: 89–102.

30 Reeves RA, Leenen FH, Joyner CD. Reproducibility of nurse-measured, exercise and ambulatory blood pressure and echocardiographic left ventricular mass in borderline hypertension. *J Hypertens* 1992; **10**: 1249–56.

31 Pickering TG. Clinical applications of ambulatory blood pressure monitoring: the white coat syndrome. *Clin Invest Med* 1991; **14**: 212–17.

32 Gosse P, Promax H, Durandet P, Clementy J. "White coat" hypertension. No harm for the heart. *Hypertension* 1993; **22**: 766–70.

33 Perloff D, Sokolow M, Cowan R. The prognostic value of ambulatory blood pressure monitoring in treated hypertensive patients. *J. Hypertens* 1991; **9** (Suppl.): S33–40.

34 Raftery EB. Direct versus indirect measurement of blood pressure. *J Hypertens* 1991; **9** (Suppl.): S10–12.

35 Omboni S, Ravogli A, Parati G, Zanchetti A, Mancia G. Prognostic value of ambulatory blood pressure monitoring. *J Hypertens* 1991; **9** (Suppl.): S25–8.

36 National High Blood Pressure Education Program Working Group. Report on ambulatory blood pressure monitoring. *Arch Intern Med* 1990; **150**: 2270–80.

37 Krakoff LR. Ambulatory blood pressure monitoring can improve cost-effective management of hypertension. *Amer J Hypertens* 1993; **6**: 220–4S.

38 West JNW, Townsend JN, Davies P *et al.* Effect of unrestricted activity on accuracy of ambulatory blood pressure measurement. *Hypertension* 1991; **18**: 593–7.

39 Cox J, Amery A, Clement D *et al.* Twenty-four hour blood pressure monitoring in the SystEuro Trial. *Ageing Clin Exp Res* 1992: **4**: 85–91.

40 Jern S, Hansson L, Hedner T. Ambulatory blood pressure – defining normalcy of a very variable variable. *Blood pressure* 1995; **4**: 264–5.

41 Staessen J, Fagard R, Lijnen P, Thijs L, van Hoof R, Amery A. Reference values for ambulatory blood pressure: a meta-analysis. *J Hypertens* 1990; **8** (Suppl.): S57–64.

42 Baumgart P, Walger P, Jurgens U, Rahn KH. Reference data for ambulatory blood pressure monitoring: what results are equivalent to the established limits of office blood pressure? *Klin Wochenschr* 1990; **68**: 723–7.

43 Broadhurst P, Brigden G, Dasgupta P, Lahiri A, Raftery EB. Ambulatory intra-arterial blood pressure in normal subjects. *Amer Heart J* 1990; **120**: 160–6.

44 Mallion JM, De Gaudemaris R, Siche JP, Maitre A, Pitiot M. Day and night blood pressure values in normotensive and essential hypertensive subjects assessed by twenty-four-hour ambulatory monitoring. *J Hypertens* 1990; **8** (Suppl.): S49–55.

45 Palatini P, Pessina AC. A new approach to define the upper normal limits of ambulatory blood pressure. *J Hypertens* 1990; **8** (Suppl.): S65–70.

46 Baumgart P. Long-term ambulatory blood pressure monitoring: what is normal?. *Z Kardiol* 1991; **80** (Suppl.1): 29–32.

47 Cesana G, De Vito G, Ferrario M *et al.* Ambulatory blood pressure normalcy: the PAMELA Study. *J Hypertens* 1991; **9** (Suppl.): S17–23.

48 Fotherby MD, Critchley D, Potter JF. Effect of hospitalization on conventional and 24-hour blood pressure. *Age Ageing* 1995; **24**: 25–9.

49 Lee DR, Swift CG, Jackson SH. Twenty-four-hour ambulatory blood pressure monitoring in healthy elderly people: reference values. *Age Ageing* 1995; **24**: 91–5.

50 Bachmann K, Wortmann A, Engels G. Ambulatory invasive and noninvasive blood pressure monitoring. *Herz* 1989; **14**: 232–7.

51 Trazzi S, Mutti E, Frattola A, Imholz B, Parati G, Mancia G. Reproducibility of non-invasive and intra-arterial blood pressure monitoring: implications for studies on antihypertensive treatment. *J Hypertens* 1991; **9**: 115–19.

52 Pickering TG. The role of ambulatory monitoring in reducing the errors associated with blood pressure measurement. *Herz* 1989; **14**: 214–20.

53 Zurmann J. Technical and methodologic aspects of ambulatory long-term blood pressure monitoring systems. *Herz* 1989; **14**: 205–13.

54 Schwan A. Postural effects on diastolic blood pressure are differently recorded by a non-invasive ambulatory blood pressure monitor and a standard auscultatory device. *Clin Physiol* 1993; **13**: 621–9.

55 Degaute JP, van de Borne P, Kerkhofs M, Dramaix M, Linkowski P. Does non-invasive ambulatory blood pressure monitoring disturb sleep? *J Hypertens* 1992; **10**: 879–85.

56 Schwan A, Eriksson G. Effect on sleep – but not on blood pressure – of nocturnal non-invasive blood pressure monitoring. *J Hypertens* 1992; **10**: 189–94.

57 Mancia G, Omboni S, Parati G, Trazzi S, Mutti E. Limited reproducibility of hourly blood pressure values obtained by ambulatory blood pressure monitoring: implications for studies on antihypertensive drugs. *J Hypertens* 1992; **10**: 1531–5.

58 Mora Macia J, Ocon Pujadas J, Ros Martrat T, del Rio Perez G. The continuous recording of ambulatory arterial pressure. The value of monitoring 4-hour subperiods. *Rev Clin Esp* 1990; **187**: 10–12.

59 Germano G, Caparra A, Valentino S, Coia F, Federico L, Santucci A. A validation of the data obtained with the simultaneous recording of blood pressure and the 24-hour electrocardiogram. *Cardiologia* 1993; **38**: 383–92.

60 O'Brien E, O'Malley K. Twenty-four-hour ambulatory blood pressure monitoring: a review of validation data. *J Hypertens* 1990; **8** (Suppl.): S11–16.

61 Coats AJ, Clark SJ, Conway J. Analysis of ambulatory blood pressure data. *J Hypertens* 1991; **9** (Suppl.): S19–21.

62 Streitberg B, Meyer-Sabellek W. Smoothing twenty-four-hour ambulatory blood pressure profiles: a comparison of alternative methods. *J Hypertens* 1990; **8** (Suppl.): S21–7.

63 Hansen KW, Ørskov H. A plea for consistent reliability in ambulatory blood pressure monitors: a reminder. *J Hypertens* 1992; **10**: 1313–15.

64 Floras JS. Will knowing the variability of ambulatory blood pressure improve clinical outcome? An additional consideration in the critical evaluation of this technology. *Clin Invest Med* 1991; **14**: 231–40.

65 Sheps SG. Cost considerations of ambulatory blood pressure monitoring. *J Hypertens* 1990; **8** (Suppl): S29–31.

66 Krakoff LR, Schechter C, Fahs M, Andre M. Ambulatory blood pressure monitoring: is it cost-effective? *J Hypertens* 1991; **9** (Suppl): S28–30.

67 Consensus document on non-invasive ambulatory blood pressure monitoring. The Scientific Committee. *J Hypertens* 1990; **8** (Suppl.): S135–40.

68 Pickering TG, O'Brien E, O'Malley K. Second international consensus meeting on twenty-four-hour ambulatory blood pressure measurement: consensus and conclusions. *J Hypertens* 1991; **9** (Suppl 8.): S2–6.

69 O'Brien E, Cox J, O'Malley K. The role of twenty-four-hour ambulatory blood pressure measurement in clinical practice. *J Hypertens* 1991; **9** (Suppl 8.): S63–5.

70 Thibonnier M. Ambulatory blood pressure monitoring. When is it warranted? *Postgrad Med* 1992; **91**: 263–74.

71 Mancia G, Omboni S, Parati G, Santucciu C, Trazzi S, Ulian L. Clinical value of ambulatory blood pressure monitoring. *Amer J Hypertens* 1993; **6**: 9–13S.

72 Zeitler HP. Long-term ambulatory blood pressure monitoring in the practice of the established physician. Report of experience. *Z Kardiol* 1991; **80** (Suppl. 1): 33–6.

73 Bass MJ. Ambulatory blood pressure monitoring and the primary care physician. *Clin Invest Med* 1991; **14**: 256–9.

74 Foster C, McKinlay, S Kemp F. Making sense of ambulatory blood pressure monitoring. *Nurs Times* 1993; **89**: 33–4.

75 Kouame N, Landry F, Jette M, Tammen AT, Blumchen G. Accuracy of ambulatory blood pressure monitoring in four exercise situations. *Herz* 1989; **14**: 221–31.

76 Blanchard EB, Cornish PJ, Wittrock DA, Jaccard J, Eisele G. Effects of 24-hour ambulatory blood pressure monitoring on daily activities. *Health Psychol* 1990; **9**: 647–52.

77 Dimsdale JE, Coy TV, Ancoli-Israel S, Clausen J, Berry CC. The effect of blood pressure cuff inflation on sleep. A polysomnographic examination. *Amer J Hypertens* 1993; **6**: 888–91.

78 Pedley CF, Bloomfield RL, Colflesh MJ, Porcel MR, Novikov SV. Blood pressure monitor-induced petechiae and ecchymoses. *Amer J Hypertens* 1994; 7: 1031–2.

79 Bottini PB, Rhoades RB, Carr AA, Prisant LM. Mechanical trauma and acute neuralgia associated with automated ambulatory blood pressure monitoring. *Amer J Hypertens* 1991; **4**: 288.

Appendix A   *References concerning methods of testing ambulatory non-invasive blood pressure monitoring equipment*

80 O'Brien E, O'Malley K, Sheridan J. The need for a standardized protocol for validating non-invasive ambulatory blood pressure measuring devices. *J Hypertens* 1989; 7 (Suppl. 3): S19–20.

81 O'Brien E, Perry I, Sheridan J, Atkins N, O'Malley K. Application of cusums to ambulatory blood pressure data: a simple statistical technique for detecting trends over time. *J Hypertens* 1989; 7: 707–9.

82 O'Brien E, O'Malley K. Twenty-four-hour ambulatory blood pressure monitoring: a review of validation data. *J Hypertens* 1990; **8** (Suppl. 6): S11–S16.

83 O'Brien E, O'Malley K. Evaluation of blood pressure measuring devices with special reference to ambulatory systems. *J Hypertens* 1990; **8** (Suppl. 6): S133–9.

84 O'Brien E, Petrie J, Littler W, deSwiet M, Padfield PL, O'Malley K. The British Hypertension Society protocol for the evaluation of automated and semi-automated blood pressure measuring devices with special reference to ambulatory systems. *J Hypertens* 1990; **8**: 607–19.

85 O'Brien E, Mee F, Atkins N, O'Malley K. Validation requirements for ambulatory blood pressure measuring systems. *J Hypertens* 1991; **9** (Suppl. 8): S13–15.

86 O'Brien E, Murphy J, Tyndall A *et al*. Twenty-four-hour ambulatory blood pressure in men and women aged 17 to 80 years: the Allied Irish Bank Study. *J Hypertens* 1991; **9**: 355–60.

87 White WB. Assessment of ambulatory blood pressure recorders: accuracy and clinical performance. *Clin Invest Med* 1991; **14**: 202–11.

88 O'Brien E, Mee F, Atkins N, O'Malley K. The quest for better validation: a critical comparison of the AAMI and BHS validation protocols for ambulatory blood pressure measurement systems. *Biomed Instrum Technol* 1992; **26**: 395–9.

89 Mancia G, Parati G. Commentary on the revised British Hypertension Society protocol for evaluation of blood pressure measuring devices: a critique of aspects related to 24-hour ambulatory blood pressure measurement. *J Hypertens* 1993; **11**: 595–7.

90 O'Brien E, Petrie J, Littler W *et al*. An outline of the revised British Hypertension Society protocol for the evaluation of blood pressure measuring devices. *J Hypertens* 1993; **11**: 677–9.

91 White WB, Berson AS, Robbins C *et al*. National standard for measurement of resting and ambulatory blood pressure with automated sphygmomanometers. *Hypertension* 1993; **21**: 504–9.

Appendix B   *References concerning tests of ambulatory non-invasive blood pressure monitors*

92 Brunner HR, Des Combes BJ, Waeber B. Porchet M. Accuracy and reproducibility of ambulatory blood pressure recordings obtained with the Remler system. *J Hypertens* 1983; **1** (Suppl. 2): 291–2.

93 Gould BA, Hornung RS, Kieso HA, Altman DA, Cashman PMM, Raftery EB. Evaluation of the Remler M2000 blood pressure recorder: comparison with intraarterial blood pressure recordings both at hospital and at home. *Hypertension* 1984: **6**: 209–15.

94 Fitzgerald D, O'Donnell D, Brennan M, O'Malley K, O'Brien E. Accuracy and reliability of the Del Mar Avionics pressurometer III. *J Hypertens* 1985; **3** (Suppl. 3): S359–61.

95 Tochikubo O, Kaneko Y, Yokoi H, Yukinari Y. A new portable device for recording 24-h indirect blood pressure in hypertensive outpatients. *J Hypertens* 1985; **3** (Suppl. 3): S355–7.

96 Hope SL, Alun-Jones E, Sleight P. Validation of the accuracy of the Medilog ABP non-invasive blood pressure monitor. *J Ambulat Monit* 1988; **1**: 39–51.

 97 Phillips DI, Braithwaite J, Newcombe RG, Lazarus JH. A clinical evaluation of the Accutracker – a lightweight ambulatory blood pressure monitor. *J Hum Hypertens* 1989; **3**: 463–5.

 98 Santucci S, Cates EM, James GD, Schussel YR, Steiner D, Pickering TG. A comparison of two ambulatory blood pressure monitors, the Del Mar Avionics Pressurometer IV and the Spacelabs 90202. *Amer J Hypertens* 1989; **2**: 797–9.

 99 White WB, Lund-Johanson P, McCabe EJ. Clinical evaluation of the Colin ABPM 630 at rest and during exercise: an ambulatory blood pressure monitor with gas-powered cuff inflation. *J Hypertens* 1989; **7**: 477–83.

100 White WB, Lund-Johanson P, McCabe EJ, Omvik P. Clinical evaluation of the Accutracker II ambulatory blood pressure monitor: assessment of performance in two countries and comparison with sphygmomanometry and intra-arterial blood pressure at rest and during exercise. *J Hypertens* 1989; **7**: 967–75.

101 Appel LJ, Whelton PK, Seidler AJ, Patel AR, Klag MJ. The accuracy and precision of the Accutracker ambulatory blood pressure monitor. *Amer J Epidemiol* 1990; **132**: 343–54.

102 Hillman D, Otsuka K, Halberg F. Ambulatory blood pressure monitor and 'analyzer'. *Chronobiologia* 1990; **17**: 305–13.

103 Imai Y, Abe K, Sasaki S *et al.* Determination of clinical accuracy and nocturnal blood pressure pattern by new portable device for monitoring indirect ambulatory blood pressure. *Amer J Hypertens* 1990; **3**: 293–301.

104 James GD, Yee LS, Cates EM, Schlussel YR, Pecker MS, Pickering TG. A validation study of the instromedix Baro-Graf QD home blood pressure monitor. *Amer J Hypertens* 1990; **3**: 717–20.

105 Jamieson MJ, Fowler G, MacDonald TM *et al.* Bench and ambulatory field evaluation of the A&D TM-2420 automated sphygmomanometer. *J Hypertens* 1990; **8**: 599–605.

106 Jyothinagaram SG, Watson D, Padfield PL. Suntech Accutracker ambulatory blood pressure monitor – clinical validation. *J Ambulat Monit* 1990; **3**: 63–7

107 Meyer-Sabellek W, Schulte KL, Gotzen R. Non-invasive ambulatory blood pressure monitoring: technical possibilities and problems. *J Hypertens* 1990; **8** (Suppl.): S3–10.

108 Modesti PA, Gensini GF, Brogi E, Neri Serneri GG. Clinical evaluation of a novel ambulatory automatic blood pressure monitoring system. *Angiology* 1990; **41**: 855–61.

109 Northcote RJ, McKillop G, Wosormu D, Kesson E, Brown JJ. Accutracker: evaluation of a new ambulatory blood pressure monitor. *Amer J Noninvasive Cardiol* 1990; **4**: 276–81.

110 O'Brien E, Mee F, Atkins N, O'Malley K. Accuracy of the Del Mar Avionics Pressurometer IV determined by the British Hypertension Society protocol. *J Hypertens* 1991; **9**: 567–8.

111 Radaelli A, Coats AJS, Clark R, Bird R, Sleight P. The effects of posture and activity on the accuracy of blood pressure recording: a validation of the Oxford Medilog system. *J Ambulat Monit* 1990; **3**: 155–61.

112 White WB, Lund-Johanson P, Omvik P. Assessment of four ambulatory blood pressure monitors and measurements by clinicians versus intrarterial blood pressure at rest and during exercise. *Am J Cardiol* 1990; **65**: 60–6.

113 Barthelemy JC, Geyssant A, Auboyer C, Antoniadis A, Berruyer J, Lacour JR. Accuracy of ambulatory blood pressure determination: a comparative study. *Scand J Clin Lab Invest* 1991; **51**: 461–6.

114 Clark S, Fowlie S, Coats A *et al.* Ambulatory blood pressure monitoring: validation of the accuracy and reliability of the TM-2420 according to the AAMI recommendation. *J Hum Hypertens* 1991; **5**: 77–82.

115 Clark S, Hofmeyr GL, Coats AJS Redman CWG. Ambulatory blood pressure monitoring during pregnancy: validation of the TM-2420 monitor. *Obstet Gynecol* 1991; **77**: 152–5.

116 Conway J. Bench and ambulatory field evaluation of the A&D TM-2420 automated sphygmomanometer. *J Hypertens* 1991; **9**: 577–8.

117 Eidemak I, Hoegholm A, Kristensen KS, Madsen NH, Nielsen HS. The new ambulatory non-invasive 24-hour blood pressure monitoring system, Takeda Medical TM 2420. Reliability and practical experiences. *Ugeskr Laeger* 1991; **153**: 335–8.

118 Groppelli A, Omboni S, Ravogli A, Villani A, Parati G, Mancia G. Validation of the SpaceLabs 90202 and 90207 devices for ambulatory blood pressure monitoring by

comparison with intra-arterial resting and ambulatory measurements. *J Hypertens* 1991; **9** (Suppl.): S334–5.

119 Hall CL, Goodfellow J, Waites J, Clinical evaluation of the Philips 5306B electronic blood pressure monitor. *J Med Eng Technol* 1991; **15**: 177–9.

120 Jamieson MJ, Petrie JC. Bench and ambulatory field evaluation of the A&D TM-2420 automated sphygmomanometer. (Reply) *J Hypertens* 1991; **9**: 578.

121 Kawarada A, Shimazu H, Ito H, Yamakoshi K. Ambulatory monitoring of indirect beat-to-beat arterial pressure in human fingers by a volume-compensation method. *Med Biol Eng Comput* 1991; **29**: 55–62.

122 O'Brien E, Atkins N, Sheridan N *et al.* Evaluation of the Accutracker II non-invasive ambulatory blood pressure recorder according to the AAMI standard. *J. Ambulat Monit* 1991; **4**: 27–33.

123 O'Brien E, Mee F, Atkins N, O'Malley K. Evaluation of the SpaceLabs 90202 non-invasive ambulatory recorder according to the AAMI Standard and BHS criteria. *J Hum Hypertens* 1991; **5**: 223–6.

124 O'Brien E, Mee F, Atkins N, O'Malley K. Accuracy of the SpaceLabs 90207 determined by the British Hypertension Society Protocol [short report]. *J Hypertens* 1991; **9**: 573–4.

125 O'Brien E, Mee F, Atkins N, O'Malley K. Accuracy of the Del Mar Avionics Pressurometer IV determined by the British Hypertension Society Protocol [short report]. *J Hypertens* 1991; **9**: 567–8.

126 O'Brien E, Mee F, Atkins N, O'Malley K. Accuracy of the Novacor DIASYS 200 determined by the British Hypertension Society Protocol [short report]. *J Hypertens* 1991; **9**: 569–70.

127 O'Brien E, Mee F, Atkins N, O'Malley K. Accuracy of the A & D TM-2420 Model 7 for ambulatory blood pressure monitoring and effect of microphone replacement. *J Ambul Monit* 1991; **4**: 281–8.

128 O'Brien E, Mee F, Atkins N, O'Malley K. Accuracy of the Takeda TM 2420/TM-2020 determined by the British Hypertension Society Protocol [short report]. *J Hypertens* 1991; **9**: 571–2.

129 O'Brien E, Mee F, Atkins N, O'Malley K. Accuracy of the SpaceLabs 90207, Novacor DIASYS 200, Del Mar Avionics Pressurometer IV and Takeda TM-2420 ambulatory systems according to British and American criteria. *J Hypertens* 1991; **9** (Suppl.): S332–3.

130 Palataini P, Penzo M, Canali C, Pessina AC. Validation of the accuracy of the A&D TM 2420 Model 7 for ambulatory blood pressure monitoring and effect of microphone replacement on performance. *J Ambulat Monit* 1991; **4**: 281–8.

131 Parati G, Groppelli A, Omboni S, Trazzi S, Frattola A, Mancia G. Testing the accuracy of blood pressure monitoring devices in ambulatory conditions. *J Hypertens* 1991; **9** (Suppl.): S7–9.

132 Raja KM, Rothman MT, Khan ZM, Khan A. Ambulatory blood pressure monitoring evaluation of a semi-automated device. *JPMA J Pak Med Assoc* 1991; **41**: 241–3.

133 White WB, Pickering TC, Morganroth J *et al.* A multicenter evaluation of the A&D TM-2420 ambulatory blood pressure recorder. *Amer J Hypertens* 1991; **4**: 890–6.

134 Zabludowski JR, Rosenfeld JB. Validation study of two automated ambulatory blood pressure monitors – the Spacelabs and Oxford apparatuses. *Isr J Med Sci* 1991; **27**: 95–8.

135 Clark S, Fowlie S, Pannarale G, Bebb G, Coats A. Age and blood pressure measurement: experience with the TM2420 ambulatory blood pressure monitor and elderly people. *Age Ageing* 1992; **21**: 398–403.

136 Groppelli A, Omboni S, Parati G, Mancia G. Evaluation of non-invasive blood pressure monitoring devices SpaceLabs 90202 and 90207 versus resting and ambulatory 24-hour intra-arterial blood pressure. *Hypertension* 1992; **20**: 227–232.

137 Harrison DW, Crews WD Jr. The Takeda Model UA-751 blood pressure and pulse rate monitor. *Biomed Instrum Technol* 1992; **26**: 325–7.

138 Hoegholm A, Eidemak I, Kristensen KS, Bang LE, Madsen NH. Clinical evaluation of the Takeda Medical (A & D) TM 2420 ambulatory blood pressure monitor. Practical experience and comparison with direct and indirect measurements. *Scand J Clin Lab Invest* 1992; **52**: 261–8.

141

139 Imai Y, Sasaki S, Minami N *et al.* The accuracy and performance of the A&D TM 2421, a new ambulatory blood pressure monitoring device based on the cuff-oscillometric method and the Korotkoff sound technique. *Amer J Hypertens* 1992; 5: 719–26.

140 Mora-Macia J, Ocon Pujadas J. Validation of a model of an automatic device for the ambulatory monitoring of blood pressure: the Spacelabs 5200. *Med Clin (Barc)* 1992; 98: 321–4.

141 O'Brien E, Mee F, Atkins N, O'Malley K. Short report: accuracy of the CH-Druck/ Pressure Scan ERKA ambulatory blood pressure measuring system determined by the British Hypertension Society Protocol. *J Hypertens* 1992; 10: 1283–4.

142 O'Brien E, Mee F, Atkins N, O'Malley K. Short report: accuracy of the Profilomat ambulatory blood pressure measuring system determined by the British Hypertension Society Protocol. *J Hypertens* 1992; 10: 1285–6.

143 Schmidt TF, Wittenhaus J, Steinmetz TF, Piccolo P, Lupsen H. Twenty-four-hour ambulatory noninvasive continuous finger blood pressure measurement with PORTAPRES: a new tool in cardiovascular research. *J Cardiovasc Pharmacol* 1992; 19 (Suppl. 6): S117–45.

144 Aitken HA, Todd JG, Kenny GN, Shennan AH, Kissane J, de Swiet M. Validation of the SpaceLabs 90207 ambulatory blood pressure monitor for use in pregnancy. *Brit J Obstet Gynaecol* 1993; 100: 904–8.

145 Bond V Jr. Bassett DR Jr, Howley ET *et al.* Evaluation of the Colin STBP-680 at rest and during exercise: an automated blood pressure monitor using R-wave gating. *Brit J Sports Med* 1993; 27: 107–9.

146 Imholz BP, Langewouters GJ, van Montfrans GA *et al.* Feasibility of ambulatory, continuous 24-hour finger arterial pressure recording. *Hypertension* 1993; 21: 65–73.

147 Kelly JJ, Hunyor SN, Ho KY. Evaluation of the reproducibility and accuracy of ambulatory blood pressure monitoring using the Takeda TM-2420 automated blood pressure monitor. *Clin Exp Hypertens* 1993; 15: 271–87.

148 Mora-Macia J, Ocon Pujadas JM, Donate Cubells T, del Rio Perez G. The evaluation of a noninvasive monitor to record ambulatory arterial pressure: the DIASYS 200 Novacor. *Med Clin (Barc)* 1993; 101: 450–4.

149 O'Brien E, Atkins N, Mee F, O'Malley K. Comparative accuracy of six ambulatory devices according to blood pressure levels. *J Hypertens* 1993; 11: 673–5.

150 O'Brien E, Mee F, Atkins N, Halligan A, O'Malley K. Accuracy of the SpaceLabs 90207 ambulatory blood pressure measuring system in normotensive pregnant women determined by the British Hypertension Society protocol. *J Hypertens* 1993; 11 (Suppl. 5): S282–3.

151 O'Brien E, Mee F, Atkins N, O'Malley K. Technical aspects of 24-hour ambulatory blood pressure monitoring. Comparative accuracy of six ambulatory systems determined by the BHS protocol. *High Blood Pressure* 1993; 2 (Suppl. 1): 76–9.

152 O'Brien E, Mee F, Atkins N, O'Malley K. Short report: accuracy of the Dinamap portable monitor, model 8100 determined by the British Hypertension Society protocol. *J Hypertens* 1993; 11: 761–3.

153 Shennan AH, Kissane J, De Swiet M. Validation of the SpaceLabs 90207 ambulatory blood pressure monitor in pregnancy. *Brit J Obstet Gynaecol* 1993; 100: 904–8.

154 Taylor R, Chidley K, Goodwin J, Broeders M, Kirby B. Accutracker II (version 30/23) ambulatory blood pressure monitor: clinical validation using the British Hypertension Society and Association for the Advancement of Medical Instrumentation standards. *J Hypertens* 1993; 11: 1275–82.

155 Bald M, Kubel S, Rascher W. Validity and reliability of 24 h blood pressure monitoring in children and adolescents using a portable, oscillometric device. *J Hum Hypertens* 1994; 8: 363–6.

156 Imai Y, Hashimoto J, Minami N *et al.* Accuracy and performance of the Terumo ES-H51, a new portable blood pressure monitor. *Amer J Hypertens* 1994; 7: 255–60.

157 Johnson AG, Nuygen TV, Day RO. Evaluation of the accuracy and reproducibility of ambulatory blood pressure monitoring in the very elderly using the Takeda TM-2420. *J Hum Hypertens* 1994; 8: 433–9.

158 Mee F, Atkins N, O'Brien E. Validation of the Nissei DS-240 ambulatory blood pressure measuring system as determined by the British Hypertension Society protocol. *J Hum Hypertens* 1994; 8: 295. (Abs.).

159 O'Brien E. Validity and reliability of 24h blood pressure monitoring in children and adolescents using a portable oscillometric device. *J Hum Hypertens* 1994; **8**: 797–8.

160 O'Brien E. Accuracy and performance of the Terumo ES-H51, a new portable blood pressure monitor. *Amer J Hypertens* 1994; **7**: 1118.

161 O'Shea JC, O'Neill A, O'Brien C, Murphy MB. Evaluation of the Tycos Quiet-Trak ambulatory pressure recorder using British Hypertension Society (BHS) protocol. *Amer J Hypertens* 1994; **7**: 118A (Abs.).

162 Tisler A, Barna I, Chatel R. Comparative study of 24-hour ambulatory blood pressure monitors with standard zero and random zero sphygmomanometers. *Orv Hetil* 1994; **135**: 1415–19.

163 White WB, Susser W, James GD *et al.* Multicenter assessment of the QuietTrak ambulatory blood pressure recorder according to the 1992 AAMI guidelines. *Am J Hypertens* 1994; **7**: 509–14.

164 O'Brien E, Atkins N. Evaluation of the accuracy and reproducibility of the Takeda TM-2429 in the elderly. *J Hum Hypertens* 1995; **9**: 205.

165 O'Brien E, Atkins N, Staessen J. State of the market. A review of ambulatory blood pressure monitoring devices. *Hypertension* 1995; **26**: 835–42.

Further reading

Pickering TG. *Ambulatory monitoring and blood pressure variability.* London: Science Press, 1991.

Waeber B, O'Brien E, O'Malley K, Brunner HR, eds. *Ambulatory blood pressure.* New York: Raven Press, 1994.

11 Home blood pressure monitoring

This chapter is concerned with the monitoring of blood pressure by patients in their own homes and with the possibilities available to others who would like to keep their blood pressures under review.[1,2]

Patients

Patients themselves are increasingly encouraged to participate in their own care. Whilst some now measure their blood pressure at intervals when on treatment or under surveillance with a view to possible treatment,[3] most still attend clinics or general practice surgeries for the measurement to be carried out. Pregnancy carries a special risk of hypertension, such that monitoring at home or in the antenatal clinic has much to commend it in those thought to be particularly susceptible.[4]

This is an area of potential growth[5] and, with proper instruction[6,7] and measures to ensure the care and accuracy of the equipment,[8] there seems no reason why patients should not monitor themselves with the same diligence and intelligence that diabetics have demonstrated for many years.[9–14] Indeed, it has been suggested that simple home monitoring of blood pressure may be preferable to ambulatory monitoring.[15] Some have advised caution in introducing home monitoring,[16,17] whereas others report satisfactory experience either with ambulatory monitoring based in the home,[18] or with both home and ambulatory monitoring.[19,20] In particular, early benefits from teletransmission of results have been reported[21] and this would appear to be an area suitable for further development. Not least, substantial cost savings have been gained for some patients without apparent detriment to their welfare.[22] The prediction of risk in hypertension from data obtained by home monitoring has been compared with that gained from random measurements and the case made for home monitoring.[23] The progress made in home blood pressure monitoring has been discussed by Pickering,[24] with special reference to ambulatory monitoring and the response to treatment.

144

Methods which merit consideration

Methods suitable for patients and others in the community need to be simple, straightforward and not unduly prone to foible and error obvious only to a skilled person. For this reason, automated blood pressure measuring devices would seem to offer a programmed approach to the measurement as such, requiring of the patient only the need to conduct it under appropriate conditions of relaxation and good positioning.

Clinical supervision

Whilst the foregoing has given encouragement to patients to measure their own blood pressures when appropriate, some guidance and supervision is necessary in that those not under treatment or supervision need to be advised of the circumstances when recourse to medical aid is necessary. More importantly, patients must continue to be reviewed periodically when conducting their own routine surveillance. Such visits, to the clinic, general practitioner or practice nurse, or by the community nurse, serve to remind the patient of the need to maintain measurements, to ensure consistency, and to have faulty or broken instruments repaired.

The general population

The present position

Paradoxically, many of the public who are not patients have responded to press coverage by purchasing their own instruments and using them regularly. We cannot be sure of the degree of familiarisation they receive when sold the devices, but many take the results they produce very seriously.

Possible developments

It is likely that the practice of self-surveillance will extend as the public becomes better informed about hypertension and its sequelae. Whether this trend will provide a platform for large-scale epidemiological studies remains to be seen.

145

Training/information required by lay users

- The basic objectives of the instrument
- The use of the controls
- The care of the cuff and the method of its application
- An appreciation of the display and/or hard-copy output
- Explanation of possible errors and their manifestation or indication
- What to do if a fault develops or the user is otherwise in need of help
- The name, address and telephone number of the repair/maintenance agent

---

Complications

Apart from the risk of hypochondria in the not-at-risk population, perhaps the only significant hazard associated with automated blood pressure measuring devices concerns those which can be set to make repeated measurements. Here, the risk of sustained vascular occlusion or intermittent occlusion, with insufficient time for arterial reperfusion and/or venous drainage, is very real as the frequency of readings increases. In hospital practice, the problem is well recognised in neonates, infants, and small children, where it has on occasion produced disastrous ischaemia. Small children and infants may not be in a position to communicate distress, so that the problem may only be recognised after damage has been inflicted. However, injury may also occur in adults. Compartment syndrome[25] and nerve injury have occurred.[26,27] The frequency of readings required in the monitoring of blood pressure in pre-eclampsia requires that especial care be exercised.[28]

Training

The moral, as always, is to insist on proper instruction by a suitably qualified person, who will inform the user of this serious potential hazard. Training to the required level of competence is essential, whatever the status of the individual and however "trivial" the procedure may seem to the uninitiated. The hazards of over-inflation and too frequent repetition of measurements need to be stressed. O'Brien has given advice to prospective home users on the significance of having been diagnosed as suffering from hypertension.[29]

Protocols

In such circumstances, protocols suitable for lay users would appear to have clear advantages.

Clear instructions

Given that the respondents will generally have no connection with the health field, it is a *sine qua non* that any instructions be written with the lay person in mind; that they should be clear, concise and unambiguous and presented attractively, and in a format that lends itself to easy reading and assimilation, using diagrams where appropriate.

Apparatus

For most applications outside hospitals and general practice premises, it seems likely that the best choices would be compact, rugged instruments, preferably with hard-copy output or a cumulative memory with printing or uploading facilities. Hard copy of repeated estimations has the advantage of revealing to the patient inconsistency in readings and the need for extra care and, if the patient does not detect such aberrations, convey the same message to anyone who subsequently examines or analyses it.

Commissioning

At present, blood pressure measuring devices are available from a wide variety of sources. Besides normal NHS and other approved sources of supply, they are available from shops and small distributors by direct purchase and mail order. It is not certain that all purchasers will get the instruction they need to get the greatest benefit from the apparatus. General practitioners and community nurses are a potential source of sound advice to intending purchasers, who should perhaps be encouraged to seek such advice. Guidance on this matter has been given by the Medical Devices Agency.[30,31]

Several authors have commented on the methodology appropriate to the testing of blood pressure apparatus consistent with home use.[32-35]

Reports of some devices which have been tested are listed in the Appendix to this chapter and are in approximately chronological order.[36-52] Reports cited by Evans *et al.*[51] and by O'Brien *et al.*[54] and also listed, are intended for lay users of such equipment.[55-58]

Preventative maintenance and running care

There is frequently contention about who is responsible for a device supplied by a hospital when the patient takes it into the community. Again, good advice has been forthcoming from the Medical Devices Agency.[30,31] Manufacturers and suppliers of the more elaborate automated devices usually offer a maintenance contract, whilst many portable automated instruments now have a high degree of reliability and, in any case, when faulty, demonstrate bizarre behaviour discernible by the user or simply fail completely. Thus, running care other than reasonable care when actually using them is probably sufficient.

Care of the equipment in the home

Equipment intended only for the home should be kept safe from inadvertent damage and in an environment suitable for its components. Generally speaking, the usual admonition to "store in a cool dry place" will suffice, with a rider stating the extremes of storage temperatures.

1 Burch GE. A sphygmomanometer in every home. *Am Heart J* 1972; **84**: 710.
2 Burch GE. Of recording your own blood pressure. *Am Heart J* 1975; **89**: 813–14.
3 Kleinert HD, Harshfield GA, Pickering TG, *et al.* What is the value of home blood pressure measurements in patients with hypertension? *Hypertension* 1984; **6**: 574–8.
4 Smith CV, Selig CL, Rayburn WF, Yi PF. Reliability of compact electronic blood pressure monitors for hypertensive pregnant women. *J Reprod Med* 1990; **35**: 399–401.
5 Hahn LP, Folsom AR, Sprafka JM, Prineas RJ. Prevalence and accuracy of home sphygmomanometers in an urban population. *Am J Public Health* 1987; 77: 1459–61.
6 Hunt JC, Frohlich ED, Moser M, Rocella EJ, Keighley EA. Devices used for self-measurement of blood pressure: revised statement of the National High Blood Pressure Education Program. *Arch Intern Med* 1985; **145**: 2231–45.
7 Kelly PL, Harrison DW. Home blood pressure monitoring: a survey of potential users. *Biomed Instrum Technol* 1994; **28**: 32–6. (Erratum appears in *Biomed Instrum Technol* 1994; **28**: 135.)
8 Nash CA. Ensuring the accuracy of digital sphygmomanometers for home use. *Mayo Clin Proc* 1994; **69**: 1006–10.
9 Burns-Cox GJ, Rees JR, Wilson RSE. Pilot study of home measurement of blood pressure by hypertensive patients. *BMJ* 1975; **iii**: 80.
10 Carnahan JE, Nugent CA. The effects of self-monitoring by patients on the control of hypertension. *Am J Med Sci* 1975; **269**: 69–73.
11 Editorial. Home blood pressure recording. *Lancet* 1975; **i**: 259–60.
12 Haynes RB, Sackett DL. Improvement of medication compliance in uncontrolled hypertension. *Lancet* 1976; **i**: 1265–8.
13 Johnson AL, Taylor DW, Sackett DL, Dunnett CW, Shimuzu AG. Self blood pressure recording in the management of hypertension. *Can Med Assoc J* 1978; **119**: 1034–9.
14 Steiner RA, Lüscher T, Siegenthaler W, Vetter W. Semi-automatic measurement of blood pressure – how reliable is it? *Deutsch Med Wochenschr* 1980; **52**: 1801–6.

15 Aylett MJ. Ambulatory or self blood pressure measurement? Improving the diagnosis of hypertension. *Fam Pract* 1994; **11**: 197–200.

16 Aberg H, Aberg K. Caution needed when evaluating blood pressure measurement taken in the home. *Lakartidningen* 1991; **88**: 1290–3.

17 Sheps SG. Finding the right role for home blood pressures. *Cleve Clin J Med* 1991; **58**: 61–3.

18 Os I, Eide I, Kjeldsen SE, Westheim A, Nordby G. Ambulatory non-invasive 24-hour blood pressure measurement – do we need it? *Tidsskr Nor Laegeforen* 1991; **111**: 2280–2.

19 Vetter W, Feltkamp H. Ambulatory blood pressure monitoring *vs.* blood pressure self monitoring. *Z Kardiol* 1991; **80** (Suppl. 1): 49–51.

20 Zachariah PK, Sheps SG, Smith RL. Clinical use of home and ambulatory blood pressure monitoring. *Mayo Clin Proc* 1989; **64**: 1436–46.

21 Vidt DG, Bolen K, Gifford RW Jr, Medendorp SV. The Telelab personal blood pressure transmitter: accurate and reliable home monitoring for hypertensive patients. *Cleve Clin J Med* 1991; **58**: 28–32.

22 Soghikian K, Casper SM, Fireman BH *et al.* Home blood pressure monitoring. Effect on use of medical services and medical care costs. *Med Care* 1992; **30**: 855–65.

23 Russo GE, Torre MC, Tosco U, Caramiello MS, Russo R, Scarpellini MG. Monitored and random arterial blood pressure as prediction of biological risk. Comparison with domiciliary self-measurement. *Ann Ital Med Int* 1990; **5**: 106–11.

24 Pickering T. Ambulatory blood pressure monitoring: an historical perspective. *Clin Cardiol* 1992; **15** (Suppl. 2): II3–5.

25 Vidal P, Sykes PJ, O'Shaughnessy M, Craddock K. Compartment syndrome after use of an automatic arterial pressure monitoring device. *Br J Anaesth* 1993; **71**: 902–4. (Erratum appears in *Br J Anaesth* 1994; **72**: 738).

26 Sy WP. Ulnar nerve palsy possibly related to use of automatically cycled blood pressure cuff. *Anesth Analg* 1981; **60**: 687–8.

27 Bickler OE, Schapera A, Bainton CR. Acute radial nerve injury from use of an automatic blood pressure monitor. *Anesthesiology* 1990; **73**: 186–8.

28 Quinn M. Automated blood pressure measurement devices: a potential source of morbidity in preeclampsia? *Am J Obstet* Gynecol 1994; **170**: 1303–7.

29 O'Brien, O'Malley K. *High blood pressure: what it means for you and how to control it.* London: MacDonald & Co., 1987.

Advice on choice, use and maintenance

30 Health Equipment Information No. 98. *Management of medical equipment and devices.* Medical Devices Directorate. London: Department of Health, 1991.

31 *The report of the Expert Working Group on alarms on clinical monitors.* London, Medical Devices Agency, 1995: pp 11–23.

Appendix

References concerning evaluation of equipment test procedures

32 Berkson DM, Whipple IT, Shireman L, Brown H, Raynor W, Shelelle RG. Evaluation of an automated blood pressure measuring device intended for public use. *Am J Public Health* 1979; **69**: 473–9.

33 Hassler CR, Lutz GA, Linebaugh R, Cunnings KD. Identification and evaluation of non-invasive blood pressure measuring techniques. *Toxicol Appl Pharmacol* 1979; **47**: 193–201.

34 Leth A, Christian B, Schnohr P, Bruun E, Moller L, Holmkjaer P. Testing of equipment for home blood pressure reading. *Acta Med Scand* 1982; **670** (Suppl.): 85–8.

35 Carroll KK, Latman NS. Evaluation of electronic, digital blood pressure monitors: Failure rates and accuracy. *Med Instrum* 1984; **18**: 263–6.

References concerning tests of blood pressure monitors suitable for home use

36 Hochberg HM, Salomon H. Accuracy of an automated ultra-sound blood pressure monitor. *Curr Ther Res* 1971; **13**: 129–38.

37 Labarthe DR, Hawkins CM, Remington RD. Evaluation of performance of selected devices for measuring blood pressure. *Am J Cardiol* 1973; **32**: 546–53.

38 Edwards RC, Goldberg AD, Bannister R, Raftery EB. The infrasound blood pressure recorder, a clinical evaluation. *Lancet* 1976; **i**: 398–400.

39 Hobbler SW, Oesterle B, Early H. Evaluation of a new automatic device for taking and recording blood pressure. *J Lab Clin Med* 1976; **88**: 826–33.

40 Ramsay LE, Nicholls MG, Boyle P. The Elag-Kohn automatic blood pressure recorder, a clinical appraisal. *Br Heart J* 1977; **77**: 795–8.

41 Cienciala T, Kocjan A. Measurement of the arterial blood pressure with electronic device Visomat 3003. *Wiad Lek* 1978; **xxxi**: 866–8.

42 Harshfield GA, Pickering TG, Laragh JH. A validation of the Del Mar Avionics ambulatory blood pressure system. *Ambul Electrocardiogr* 1979; **1**: 7–12.

43 Savage JM, Dillon MJ, Taylor JFN. Clinical evaluation and comparison of the infrasonde and mercury sphygmomanometer in measurement of blood pressure in children. *Arch Dis Childr* 1979; **54**: 184–9.

44 Tam G. A comparison of two electronic sphygmomanometers with the traditional mercury type. *Nursing Times* 1979; **i**: 880–5.

45 Clement DL, De Pue N, Packet L, Bobelyn M, Van Maele GO. Performance of noninvasive ambulatory blood pressure recordings. *J Hypertens* 1983; **1** (Suppl. 2): 296–8.

46 Fitzgerald DL, O'Callaghan WG, McQuaid R, O'Malley K, O'Brien E. Accuracy and reliability of two indirect ambulatory blood pressure recorders: Remler M2000 and Cardiodyne Sphygmolog. *Br Heart J* 1982; **48**: 572–9.

47 Bassein L, Borghi C, Costa FV, Strocchi E, Mussi A, Ambrosioni E. Comparison of three devices for measuring blood pressure. *Statist Med* 1985; **4**: 361–8.

48 Steiner R, Luscher T, Boerlin H-J, Siegenthaler W, Vetter W. Clinical evaluation of semiautomatic blood pressure evices for self-recording. *J Hypertens* 1985; **3** (Suppl.): 23–5.

49 Pickering TG, Cvetkovski B, James GD. An evaluation of electronic recorders for self-motivation of blood pressure. *J Hypertens* 1986; **4** (Suppl. 5): S328–30.

50 Ornstein S, Markert G, Litchfield L, Zemp L. Evaluation of DINAMAP blood pressure monitor in an ambulatory primary care setting. *J Fam Pract* 1988; **26**: 517–21.

51 Evans CE, Haynes RB, Goldsmith CH, Clewson SA. Home blood pressure-measuring devices: a comparative study of accuracy. *J Hypertens* 1989; **7**: 133–42.

52 O'Brien E, Atkins N, Mee F, O'Malley K. Inaccuracy of seven popular sphygmomanometers for home-measurement of blood pressure. *J Hypertens* 1990; **8**: 621–34.

53 Salaita K, Whelton PK, Seidler AJ. A community-based evaluation of the Vita-Stat automatic blood pressure recorder. *Am J Hypertens* 1990; **3**: 366–72.

54 O'Brien E, Mee F, Atkins N, O'Malley K. Accuracy of the Dinamap portable monitor, Model 8100, determined by the British Hypertension Society protocol. *J Hypertens* 1993; **11**: 761–3.

150

References concerning reports on home blood pressure monitors directed at home users themselves

55 Consumer Reports. *Blood pressure kits.* March 1979.
56 Canadian Consumer. *Pressure point.* July 1982: 23–6.
57 Canadian Consumer. *Electronic blood pressure monitors.* February 1987: 21–4.
58 Keep your blood pressure down. *Which?* August 1989, 372–5.

12 Pulse monitoring

The "finger-on-the-pulse" is the time-honoured indication of anaesthetic vigilance. In the operating theatre, as elsewhere, not only can the rate of the heart be estimated, but its character, strength, volume, and rhythm may be appreciated, as can its presence or absence. Moreover, there are circumstances in which monitoring equipment is not provided or, if provided, is functioning imperfectly or not at all. Further, in emergency or domestic situations, before equipment is applied to the patient, much may be gleaned from careful taking of the pulse.

Why, then, should we monitor the pulse automatically? Although monitoring cannot yet replace clinical appraisal, it is a substantial weapon in the clinical armamentarium. It often frees the hands of the user who may have other tasks to perform, a consideration of some importance in anaesthesia and critical care nursing. Properly set alarms also allow the clinician or nurse engaged in demanding tasks or supervising specific therapeutic equipment to ignore normal data, whilst having a satisfactory expectation of being alerted to the abnormal. The pulse monitor, although perhaps a humble monitoring instrument, exemplifies the principle well.

Early pulse monitors were usually finger plethysmographs,[1–3] photoelectric blood densitometers (a bulb or other light source shining

---

Pulse monitors

Advantages

- May be compact and portable
- Often battery-operated
- Under good conditions, amplitude displays give a true indication of perfusion
- Often useful in emergencies

Disadvantages

- Information on only one circulatory variable
- Only as good as the sensor and its attachment
- May perform poorly when information most needed (e.g. in poor perfusional "shock" states)
- Under some conditions rate and/or amplitude displays may be misleading

---

Some operating principles of pulse monitors

- Plethysmography
- Photoelectric densitometry (light source and sensor)
- Crystal microphone
- Piezoelectric crystal
- Ultrasound detection (see Chapter 13)

---

through the pulp of the finger and sensed by a photoelectric cell),[4-6] crystal microphones[7,8] or piezoelectric crystal sensors[9,10] applied to a digit or, sometimes, more proximally on a limb. They generated pulsatile electrical signals such as illuminated an audible or visible pulse indictor, activated a galvanometer where the indicating needle traversed a scale, or a fed a digital counter. An early commercial example was the Cotel-Keating pulse monitor.[7] Thus, indication (audible or visible) could be given of pulse frequency, whilst the needle working against a scale might convey information related to the volume of the pulse. This latter information could be used in two ways: to follow the changes in pulse volume; and to ascertain whether or not the sensor was properly applied. A constant problem, as with current tonometers and plethysmographs, was detachment or displacement of the sensor. On the other hand, the devices were simple and usually, since they were generally battery-powered, neat, convenient, and portable. Sara and Shanks specifically examined plethysmographic pulse monitoring but, in passing, described several other types.[11]

Applications have included evaluation peripheral vascular disease in the elderly,[12] the effectiveness of sympathetic blocks,[13,14] and the suitability of the radial artery for cannulation.[15] Applications of pulse monitoring in general anaesthesia have been concerned with the onset and depth of anaesthesia,[16] feed-back control of halothane anaesthesia,[17,18] and the monitoring of dental anaesthesia.[19]

Digital pulse monitors operating on most of the principles listed in the box rely on good local perfusion and are most effective when the digit is warm and the patient well hydrated and not vasoconstricted. Conversely, they tend to perform poorly in cold and shocked patients, when it matters most. The early models incorporating qualitative analogue meter displays were highly susceptible to subjective interpretation.[20] Complications have arisen from local pressure effects.[8,21]

Pulse monitors of this kind are rarely seen nowadays, the principal reason being that the information given by them may so easily be derived from other monitoring signals already being gathered from the patient. Pulse frequency, for example, is often derived from the QRS-wave of the

153

Conditions for pulse monitoring

Advantageous

- Good cardiac output
- Good state of hydration
- Warm extremities
- Vasodilatation

Disadvantageous

- Poor cardiac output
- Poor state of hydration
- Cold extremities
- Vasoconstriction

electrocardiogram or from the peak voltage of the signal representing an arterial pressure wave. Alternatively, pulse frequency may be inferred from the visual characteristics of the ECG waveform. Hence, a separate instrument is regarded as unnecessary and unduly space-occupying. The declining use of pulse monitors in clinical practice stands in contrast to the growing popularity of pulse frequency counters promoted as bio-feedback devices in various forms of alternative therapies and in sports medicine.

Pulse frequency indications derived from other information signals must be interpreted with care.

ECG-derived signals

Where the heart rate is derived from the ECG signal, errors may arise when other parts of the ECG waveform are of an amplitude close to that of the R-wave and are duly spuriously detected and counted. Bifid R-waves may also be counted erroneously. Modern instruments are designed to avoid this kind of elementary error, but cannot usually eliminate the problem altogether. Arrhythmias present obvious difficulties as does a drifting electrical baseline. Careful design of the ECG monitor can minimise the untoward effects, but users should be aware of the possibilities. Thus, the displayed rate may not equate with the true heart rate and the presence of a QRS-wave does not necessarily denote that there is sufficient cardiac output for the pulse to be present. For a number of reasons, therefore, the indicated heart rate may not be that of the pulse.

Problems in pulse monitoring

Physical

- Positioning of sensor
- Dislodgement of sensor

Sources of error (rate)

- Arrhythmia
- Counting of inappropriate segments (e.g. large P- or T-waves)
- Bifid QRS waves (incorrect count)
- Bigeminy (correct, but misleading, count)
- Electrical interference

Sources of error (amplitude)

- Poor perfusion, etc.
- Loose attachment
- "Normalisation" of pulse oximeter waveform

Pressure-derived signals

Here again, all may not be what it seems, since the waveform may not have a single distinct peak amplitude or an arrhythmia may be present. Despite design features such as filtering or software intended to eliminate such confusion, the result may sometimes be erroneous. In this instance, the user often has the benefit of a visible trace on an oscilloscope screen or similar display to help validate the indicated pulse rate.

Pulse oximetry

Pulse oximeters use a similar principle to that seen in some of the earlier photoelectrical instruments, inasmuch as the optical properties of the digit and its contained blood are used in the sensing process.[22] Since the instrument seeks a peak value for its own purposes of measurement, it is a simple matter to count the peaks. As a frequency monitor, it is therefore generally satisfactory. Of more concern is the tendency for the output to be converted to a "pulse" waveform, originally conceived as a straightforward means for the user to determine whether the sensor was correctly applied and the instrument otherwise functioning properly. In order to refine this validation process, the waveform has often been artificially "normalised", i.e. it is amplified or attenuated automatically to present a waveform of ideal amplitude for appreciation during this validation exercise.

155

Unfortunately, the waveform which follows the perfusion status of the digit at the sensing site may be thought to be representing pulse amplitude, to which the signal from the sensor may, in fact, correspond reasonably closely. However, even this latter may not necessarily be the case and normalisation may give an altogether misleading impression. Manufacturers of pulse oximeters often give useful information in the instructions for the user in the operating manual and may incorporate warnings concerning the status of the waveform on accompanying displays. Nevertheless, users need to be sure that they are thoroughly familiar with their instrument before accepting displayed waveforms as quantitative information concerning the pulse. They should certainly be circumspect about mentally converting such images into pressures.

1 Burch GE, Cohn AE, Neumann C. A study by quantitative methods of the spontaneous variation in volume of the finger tip, toe tip and posterior superior portion of the pinna of resting white adults. *Am J Physiol* 1942; **136**: 433–47.
2 Burch GE, De Pasquale N. Relation of arterial pressure to spontaneous variation in digital volume. *J Appl Physiol* 1960; **15**: 23–4.
3 Hertzmann AB. Photoelectric plethysmography of the fingers and toes in man. *Proc Soc Biol Med* 1937; **37**: 529.
4 Robinson RE, Eastwood DW. Use of a photosphygmomanometer in indirect peripheral blood pressure measurement. *Anesthesiology* 1959; **20**: 704.
5 Schotz S, Bloom SS, Helmsworth FW, Dodge HC, Birkmire EC. The ear oximeter as a circulatory monitor. *Brit J Anaesth* 1959; **31**: 190–3.
6 Phelps JA, Sass DJ. A portable battery-powered instrument for visualizing the peripheral pulse wave form and pulse rate. *Anesth Analg* 1969; **48**: 582–6.
7 Keating WJ. A simple pulse indicator. *BMJ* 1952; **i**: 1188.
8 Hart RM. Pulse monitoring. *Aust Med J* 1962; **49 (1)**: 280–2.
9 Johnstone M. The effects of sedation on the plethysmogram. A radio-telemetric study of haloperidol. *Anaesthesia* 1967; **22**: 3–15.
10 Thune P. Plethysmographic recordings of skin pulses with particular reference to the piezo-electric method. I – Preliminary report. *Acta Dermatol* 1970; **50**: 27–30.
11 Sara CA, Shanks CA. The peripheral pulse monitor – a review of electrical plethysmography. *Anaesth Intens Care* 1978; **6**: 226–33.
12 Lichti EL, Keiter WF, Henzel JH, De Weese MS. Atraumatic evaluation of peripheral vascular disease in older patients. *Geriatrics* 1971; **26**: 80–5.
13 Beene TK, Eggers GW Jr. Use of pulse monitor for determining sympathetic block of the arm. *Anesthesiology* 1974; **40**: 412–14.
14 Brodsky JB. Simple method to determine the patency of the ulnar artery intra-operatively prior to radial artery cannulation. *Anesthesiology* 1975; **42**: 626–7.
15 Kim JM, Awakawa K, Von Lintel T. Use of the pulse-wave monitor as a measurement of diagnostic sympathetic block and of surgical sympathectomy. *Anesth Analg Curr Res* 1975; **54**: 289–96.
16 Johnstone M. Digital vaso-dilatation as a sign of anaesthesia. *Br J Anaesth* 1974; **46**: 414–19.
17 Beddard J. Amplitude observation during closed circuit halothane anaesthesia with the vaporiser inside the circuit. *Br J Anaesth* 1965; **37**: 354–62.
18 Suppan P. Feed-back monitoring in anaesthesia. II: Pulse rate control of halothane administration. *Br J Anaesth* 1972; **44**: 1263–71.
19 Muir VMJ. Pulse monitors in outpatient dental anaesthesia. *Anaesthesia* 1973; **28**: 312–17.
20 Eastwood DW. Monitoring the anesthetised patient (cited in). *Anesthesiology* 1970; **32**: 180.

21 Lebowitz MH. Gangrene of the finger following the use of the photoelectric plethysmograph during anaesthesia. *Anesthesiology* 1970; **32**: 164–7.
22 Moyle JBT. *Pulse oximetry.* London: BMJ Publishing Group, 1994: 108–28.

Further reading

O'Rourke MF, Kelly RP, Aviolo AP. *The arterial pulse.* Philadelphia: Lea and Febiger, 1992.

13 Doppler ultrasound monitoring, including echocardiography

Theory and physical principles

The principle described by Doppler and known as the Doppler effect concerns sound waves emitted from a particular point being reflected back when they meet the surface of a relatively dense object (Figure 13.1).[1]

The Doppler effect (Figure 13.2) depends upon wave propagation in a suitable medium. An example often quoted to illustrate the general principle of wave propagation is of the stone dropped vertically into a pond creating oscillations of the molecules of water such that ripples are produced which, in turn, appear to travel towards the periphery of the pond. In fact, it is the propagated energy which produces the oscillation along its path of propagation. The height of the ripple in relation to the level of the still pond surface is the equivalent of the *amplitude* of the wave, and the distance between the peaks of the ripples is equivalent to the *wavelength*. The ripples reach the shore at intervals corresponding to the *frequency* of oscillation of the wave. The velocity of the wave is equal to the wavelength multiplied

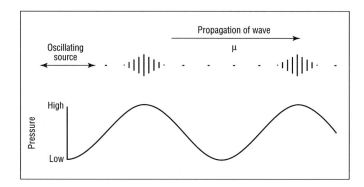

Figure 13.1 When produced by an oscillating source, a sound wave is propagated longitudinally and is characterised by zones of high pressure separated by zones of low pressure. These correspond to the contours of the pressures recorded in the transmitting medium.[3]

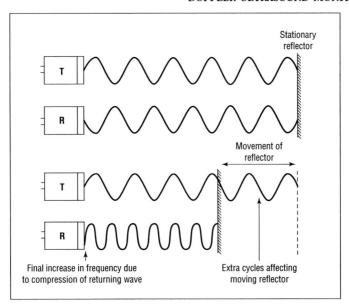

Stationary
reflector

T

R

Movement of
reflector

T

R

Final increase in frequency due
to compression of returning wave

Extra cycles affecting
moving reflector

Figure 13.2 Doppler effect. An object moving towards the transmitter encounters more cycles per second than a stationary object so that the reflected waves have a higher frequency than those from the transmitter. The increase in frequency sensed by the receiver is doubled because the reflected waves are also compressed into a shorter distance, thus decreasing their wavelength and increasing the apparent frequency further. For clarity, the incident and reflected waves are shown as parallel beams though in reality they are superimposed.[3] T = transmitter; R = receiver.

by the frequency, where the symbols for wavelength, frequency and velocity of a longitudinally propagated wave are λ, f and c, respectively. Thus:

$$\text{The velocity } (c) = \lambda \times f.$$

However, it should be noted that, in the case of sound, the oscillation is applied in the direction of propagation rather than perpendicularly to it. The result is that the wave is propagated in the direction of the applied sound oscillation. The difference between the two phenomena may be likened to that between a vibrating wire (where the oscillation is at right angles to the path of propagation) and a train of shunted railway wagons (where the buffers of a wagon strike those of the next wagon which is shunted into the next, and so on down the line of wagons).

Where sound is concerned, we speak of the *pitch* rather than the frequency, although the pitch is determined by the frequency of pulses (the number of pulses per second). As mentioned at the beginning of this chapter, sound is reflected from an identifiable surface. If the surface is approaching the sound, the reflections will increase in number per unit time so that the

159

Theoretical basis

If the frequency of the emitted signal is f_0, the wavelength is λ, and the velocity is c,

$$f_0 = \frac{c}{\lambda}$$

when the target is moving towards the source at a velocity v, the frequency of the waves hitting the target is

$$f = \frac{c+v}{\lambda}$$

but the target is also reflecting the wave back at the same frequency, so that the frequency detected by the receiver has twice that value, that is,

$$f_r = \frac{c+2v}{\lambda}$$

and the perceived increase in frequency is:

$$f_r - f_0 = \frac{c+2v}{\lambda} - \frac{c}{\lambda} = \frac{2v}{\lambda}$$

or, substituting for $\lambda = c/f_0$,

$$f_r - f_0 = \frac{2vf_0}{c}$$

Here, the resulting frequency shift is:

$$f_r - f_0 = \frac{2f_0 v \cos \theta}{c}$$

wavelength is effectively reduced and the pitch correspondingly increased.

Conversely, if the surface is receding from the sound source, the pitch will fall. Examples in daily life include the phenomenon where the pitch of the note of an approaching road vehicle apparently increases until it passes the observer and seems to decrease as the vehicle passes away, and the echo sounders used in gauging the depth of water beneath a ship.

An extension of the principle covers the circumstances in which the surface from which the sound waves are reflected is moving at an angle in relation to the source. In this latter case, the sound waves are reflected along a line at an angle θ to the line of incidence and this angle is proportional to the velocity of the moving object and its disposition (Figure 13.3). Here, the resulting frequency shift is:

$$f_r - f_0 = \frac{2f_0 v \cos \theta}{c}$$

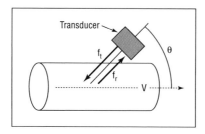

Figure 13.3 Doppler measurement of velocity is inversely related to the cosine of the angle (θ) between the Doppler transducer and blood flow velocity (see text). At angles greater than 20°, significant underestimation of velocity occurs.[2] f_t = transmitted Doppler frequency; f_r = received Doppler frequency; V = velocity of blood flow

The ideal situation is that in which the moving object travels along a plane perpendicular to the line of incidence of the sound waves. If, however, an emitter and a detector are set up as in Figure 13.3, the displacement (θ) corresponds to the velocity of the moving object.

Ultrasound sources can focus a narrow beam of ultrasound on a specific site, known as the *target*. It may also be pulsed in such a way that its duration is only a few cycles, and penetration of tissues is controlled. This feature is of fundamental importance in ultrasound tissue scanning, but only of minor importance in the cardiovascular monitoring applications we are concerned with here.

Vessel wall movement

Of much greater significance is the fact that ultrasound is reflected from junctions between tissues and between tissues and other media (Figure 13.4). This interface reflection is the basis of qualitative and quantitative estimations of flow velocity in blood vessels. If an emitter and a detector are set up as in Figure 13.5, the displacement (or angle) observed corresponds to the velocity of the moving object and may be calibrated accordingly.

Blood flow

Blood has properties that permit it to reflect sound waves. Negligible deflection occurs as the sound wave passes through the static surrounding tissues including the blood vessel wall. In practice, ultrasound has the characteristics required for satisfactory measurements to be made. In the case of blood pressure measurement, we need not know the velocity of the blood stream, but simply that there is flow that is continuous or intermittent. On this basis, devices have been designed to detect blood flow in arteries

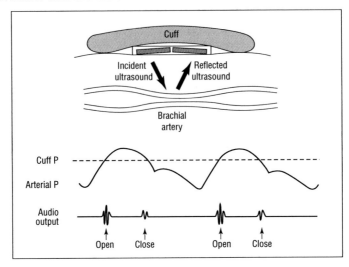

Figure 13.4 Ultrasound sphygmomanometry. Two transducer elements are placed between the cuff and the containing sheath. One of these (shown on the left) transmits a Doppler frequency to the arterial wall and the other (to the right) receives the reflected Doppler frequency. The corresponding cuff and arterial pressures are shown, as is the audio output conventionally provided with these devices and indicating relative opening and closure of the artery. [1] *and Stegall et al., J. Appl. Physiol. 1968; 25:793–98.*

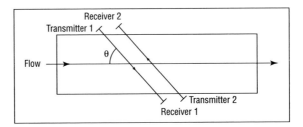

Figure 13.5 When Doppler frequencies are passed through flowing liquid, the incident ultrasound transmitted by transmitting transducer 1 and received by receiving transducer 1 makes an angle (θ) with the blood flow. Similarly, the reflected ultrasound transmitted by transmitting transducer 2 and received by receiving transducer 2 also makes an angle (θ) with the blood flow which, in this instance, is effectively in the opposite direction and, hence, yields a different value for θ. Redrawn from reflection diagram (flow).

(see Chapter 4). If the sensor is applied at the wrist or over the brachial artery, for example, there will be clear indications of the beginning of flow (at the systolic pressure), through a period of intermittent flow (or to be more accurate, intermittently changing flow velocity), and the establishment of continuous flow (ie, when the flow is no longer pulsatile) corresponding to the diastolic pressure.

162

Methods of detection

Ultrasound is generated by transducers based on the piezo-electric effect. The ceramic materials usually employed have characteristics such that the application of pressure to the crystals of the material results in the appearance of electrical charges of differing polarity on its opposing surfaces. An electrical potential difference is thus set up. In the event that the pressure applied is oscillatory in nature, the potential difference changes its polarity accordingly and the potential difference oscillates in the manner of alternating current. The emitted energy *intensity*, expressed in watts per square metre, is that crossing a unit area perpendicular to the beam. Since the *power* is the intensity multiplied by the area, the areas in the equation cancel out, leaving the power as watts, that is:

$$\text{intensity} = \frac{watts}{m^2}$$

$$\text{whilst power} = \text{intensity} \times \text{area} = \frac{watts}{m^2} \times m^2 = \text{watts}.$$

The principle has been exploited in the cartridge of record players, where the needle follows a groove in the record, alternately loading and releasing pressure on piezo-electric crystal material. The same principle is used in some crystal microphones.

The inverse of the principle may be seen in electronic paint sprays, ultrasonic drug nebulisers, and ultrasonic nebulising humidifiers, when a piezo-electric crystal is subjected to an alternating electrical current. The resultant oscillation, at the frequency of the current source, is imparted to the liquid in question, whereupon it gains energy sufficient to eject it from a nozzle.

Ultrasound transducers used in medical measurements commonly exhibit both types of behaviour and house both emitter and detector in the measurement probe. In this type, the incident beam is almost parallel to the reflected beam, so that a device constructed in this way senses only movement as such satisfactory, the angle of refraction being too small to be of value. Other types have separate emitting and receiving units, displaced such that the angle of incidence is appreciable. These types are also capable of indicating direction and velocity.

A typical schematic for an ultrasound transducer is shown in Figure 13.6.

Ultrasound is sound at a frequency above that which can be detected by the human ear. This is taken as being at a frequency about 20 kHz (although in practice most people are limited to a lower level of some

163

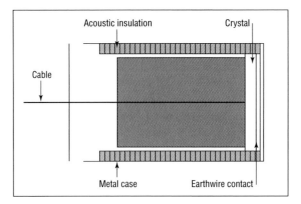

Figure 13.6 Diagram of ultrasound transducer.[3]

15 kHz, the level of auditory perception declining with age). The useful range of frequencies for medical measurement is of the order of 1–10 MHz, these values having been selected on the basis that the speed of propagation of sound through human tissues is about $15 \, \text{m s}^{-1}$ with an effective wavelength of 150 μm to 1·5 mm. So far as is known ultrasound at this frequency is without hazard in humans, although some doubt has been raised about the undesirable effects of ultrasound as used in certain obstetric investigations and the subject is still under review. We may therefore reasonably consider it to be non-invasive.

Background to clinical development

Measurement of flow in non-Newtonian fluids

As has been shown, ultrasound of a character and pulse duration such that it can be aimed at the interface between tissues can produce a reflected signal proportional to the extent of the movement at the interface. If this is at the vessel wall, it provides a means of enabling qualitative detection of that movement to be achieved. Since the movement of the vessel wall takes place in both directions, in systole and diastole, the process is repeated at the pulse frequency, so that the pulse rate may be counted electronically.

Non-Newtonian fluids, ie, those whose constituents do not flow uniformly, behave in a similar fashion. Blood is such a fluid and can be differentiated from its surroundings by ultrasound. The blood in motion, moreover, reflects ultrasound along a path at an angle to that of the incident beam, so that the beam is both reflected and refracted. As with light, scatter occurs on impact, but this is at a minimum if the incident beam is perpendicular to the target surface or interface. The value of the angular displacement (θ) of the reflected beam can be calibrated to be proportional to the velocity of blood flow in the vessel.

Apparatus

The emitter-detector transducer is admirably suited to this application. A number of commercial instruments are available. At first, their main use was the detection of venous occlusion, as in deep venous thrombosis, but they have since been used extensively in relation to other blood vessels, and especially to estimate blood flow in atheromatous arteries before and after surgical disobliteration.

Aortic flow estimation

Since the late 1960s attempts have been made to estimate blood flow in the aorta, usually as a basis for the estimation of cardiac output, in a technique sometimes referred to as aortic velography on account of the fact that it is the velocity of the blood that is sensed.[2-4] The ultrasound has been directed at the aorta at a point which is both accessible and where it encounters the least thickness of intervening tissue. A suitable site is the suprasternal notch. In early applications the ultrasound probe, when placed in the suprasternal notch, was directed towards the arch of the aorta. It is now more commonly directed at the aortic root. Besides being at a site preceding the distribution of the cardiac output to the head and upper limbs via the carotid and brachiocephalic arteries, respectively, it is more easily definable in practice.

One of the problems that may be encountered is erroneous detection of other large vessels in the vicinity, as when aiming at the aortic arch, pulmonary and braciocephalic vessels may be encountered. In the case of placement in the suprasternal notch this is less likely. It has been noted that the velocity of the blood in the pulmonary artery is less than that in the aortic root, whilst that in the brachiocephalic arteries may be greater[5] but both are in any case avoided when the suprasternal notch is chosen. The peak velocity (it is the peak velocity which is of prime interest) in the aorta in normal subjects lies in the range $0 \cdot 6$–$1 \cdot 2 \text{ m s}^{-1}$, but may be much higher in normal subjects as well as those (including some critically ill patients) in high cardiac output states.[6]

Other problems include variations in the type and depth of intervening tissue, requiring individual calibration for this reason alone, and the requirement for the cross-sectional area of the aorta at the site of measurement to be known or estimated. This latter was at first achieved radiologically, although the degree of error in the estimates proved

165

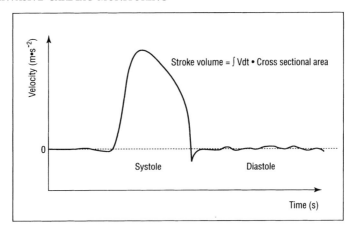

Figure 13.7 Stroke volume is calculated as the time integral of aortic velocity times aortic cross-sectional area[B].

unacceptably large for other than qualitative estimations. Nowadays the profile and hence the cross-sectional area of the aorta can be determined by a variety of advanced scanning methods with acceptable results. The flow is based on the cross-sectional area being assumed to be $\pi(d/2)^2$.

The non-invasive determination of cardiac output rests on calculation of the product of stroke volume and heart rate. Stroke volume (SV) = $V \times ET \times CSA$, where V is the average velocity of the blood in the aorta during systole, ET is the time taken for ejection of the blood and CSA is the cross-sectional area of the aorta (see Figure 13.7). The velocity and ejection time may be obtained from the ascending aorta, usually using continuous-wave Doppler emitted by a transducer in the suprasternal notch, and the cross-sectional area of the aorta by aiming pulsed Doppler from the parasternal region in the 3rd or 4th intercostal space. This two-dimensional Doppler technique can identify the near and far walls of the aortic root and enable the distance between them, the diameter, to be calculated. This assumes that the size of the aorta is synonymous with the size of the flow channel, but this is not so in aortic valvular stenosis and is confounded where there is substantial valvular regurgitation. It is probably impossible to obtain reliable results in such circumstances without continuous computation.[7]

The profile of the blood flow is clearly of importance. In humans it is thought to be "flat", that is, to be of virtually uniform velocity at the centre of the vessel and the periphery, with no effective boundary layer to cause distortions.[8] It has also been described as "plug-shaped".[9]

The ultrasound signal frequencies employed have generally been 2·5 MHz or 5 MHz and for computational purposes the velocity of sound in blood is assumed to be 15·7 m sec^{-1}, while the angle subtended by the ultrasound beam (θ) is taken as zero, such that cos θ = 1 for practical purposes. Even so, as the cosine of the angle changes little at small angles, the error introduced by slight angulation would be small.

Two forms of Doppler signal are commonly described: continuous-wave Doppler (CWD) and pulsed Doppler (PD). While CWD, as its name suggests, is continuously emitted by the ultrasound transducer, in the case of PD the signal is transmitted to the site of interest in pulses between which the transducer acts as a receiver. A significant practical difference relates to the fact that CWD interacts with any moving target at any point along the length of the beam, whereas PD allows localisation of activity to a particular point at a given distance along the beam, thereby enabling it to be focused. In the case of PD also, maximum detectable velocity decreases with increasing depth of penetration.[10] A potential drawback of PD is that there is a limit to the velocity that can be estimated reliably on account of a phenomenon known as aliasing. It is attributable to a (sinusoidal) ultrasound wave being detected in two successive samplings with a given separation which we may call x. The wavelength may therefore indeed be x, but may also be less than this, say $0.5x$, $0.33x$, $0.25x$ or some smaller fraction, depending on the number of intervening undetected waves. The waveform must therefore be subject to a sampling rate at a frequency twice that of its own or, to put it another way, aliasing will occur if the Doppler shift is greater than half the pulse repetition rate[11] or sampling frequency (the Nyquist limit).[12] The phenomenon of aliasing produces the familiar effect seen when light strobing a rotating wheel at a frequency different from that at which the spokes follow one another yields the impression of slow forward or backward rotation or, for example, when a film camera running at a particular number of frames per second similarly captures the spokes of a rotating wheel or the radial vanes of a wheel hub cap to give the same impression.

This kind of investigation is often undertaken in specialised units and the details need not concern us here. The attractions of such a method of estimating cardiac output in the critically ill patient are, however, obvious and several instruments have been introduced to cater for this need. There are, however, inherent problems arising from common features of these critically ill patients. For example, the time taken to achieve serial readings causes difficulties in monitoring patients whose cardiovascular variables are unstable, air in the mediastinum causes interference, and PEEP introduces complications in the method. Besides, the problems associated with the intervening tissues and inability to obtain reliable measurements of the cross-sectional area of the aorta, combined with difficulty in gaining convenient and stable access for the placement of the transducer, have militated against general adoption of the method in coronary care and intensive care units. The first of these is relative and can be overcome to a large extent by calibrating the instrument against the individual patient

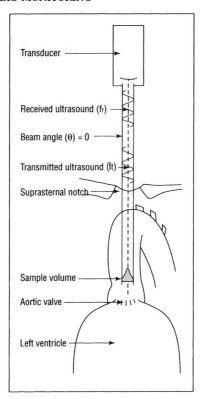

Transducer

Received ultrasound (f_r)

Beam angle (θ) = 0

Transmitted ultrasound (f_t)

Suprasternal notch

Sample volume

Aortic valve

Left ventricle

Figure 13.8 Diagram showing the principle of the Doppler method for measurement of cardiac output. Redrawn from Donovan GJ, Dobb KD, Non-invasive methods of measuring cardiac output, Intens Care Med. *1989; 13: 304–9.*

and taking a series of readings. In this connection, there appears to be no evidence that experienced operators obtain better readings (ie, that there is no learning curve).[11] The problem with the aorta is less easy to solve, not least given that the area varies with square of the diameter, so that small errors in the estimate of the diameter yield much larger errors in the area. One authority notes that a 2 mm error in the estimation of the diameter resulted in a 14% error in calculation of blood flow and many measurements had an error greater than 2 mm, while the aorta is not necessarily round at the point of measurement.[12] It has also been noted that the particular site chosen at the root, be it close to the cusps, at the sinuses of Valsalva, or elsewhere, is not of great importance as a source of error.[13,14] On the other hand, the cross-sectional area of the aorta may itself change by some 3–12% during ejection, and may therefore give rise to one of the larger errors in aortic flow (and hence cardiac output) estimation.[15]

Despite these real problems, serial cardiac output measurements using the suprasternal notch (Figure 13.8) have achieved a measure of success.

168

The technique has much to commend it as a monitoring method when access is otherwise limited, bearing in mind that the invasive methods dependent upon dye and thermal dilution techniques also have errors associated with them[16,17] and carry a small morbidity and mortality in the critically ill.[18] Good correlation with Fick methods and thermal dilution cardiac output computation has been claimed by some in adults,[7,9,19-22] with good reproducibility,[3,23,24] and in children[25] and neonates.[24] Others, however, have been unable to confirm good correlation in heart failure[26] and in other circumstances. It has been observed that there may be a better correlation with cardiac index than with cardiac output and the method has been recommended for the determination of both cardiac index and systemic vascular resistance in critically ill children.[27] Non-invasive Doppler measurement of cardiac output may be useful in establishing whether or not invasive measurements are likely to be valuable in a given patient. Huntsman[7] claimed that cardiac output measurements were possible in 85% of intensive care unit patients whether they were made by trained personnel or by nurses relatively inexperienced in the technique, and good correlation with thermal dilution cardiac output estimation has been claimed there also.[7,26,27] Moreover, the method has been shown to be of value in the monitoring of cardiac output in critically ill children.[27,28,29] In paediatric and neonatal monitoring, it is important to be aware of the effects large cardiac and great vessel shunts would have, although these are readily avoided by careful positioning of the probe, while the technique is limited in the presence of left ventricular outflow obstruction, large local shunts (as in patent ductus arteriosus), and when the aorta is on the right side and in close proximity to other vessels.[27]

Transoesophageal echocardiography (TEE)

The principle may be applied to a probe suitable for introduction into the oesophagus (Figure 13.9). The technique is known as transoesophageal echocardiography (or transesophageal echocardiography, prompting the acronym TEE). Though not altogether non-invasive, it is less so than other methods of getting close to blood vessels and may perhaps be considered minimally invasive.[30] Because of its position in the oesophagus, the probe is directed at flow in the descending aorta.

Pulsed Doppler (PD) is well suited to the application. Pulses of ultrasound are substituted for the customary continuous ultrasound and the probe acts as a receiver during the intervals between the pulses. The directional sensitivity of the device is thereby potentially improved although, as mentioned previously, pulse frequency and sampling rate must be matched so as to avoid aliasing.[11,12] CWD has also been used and refinement of transducers so that they may more readily produce two-dimensional images

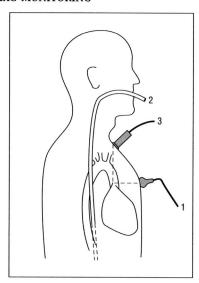

Figure 13.9 The three steps required in the measurement of cardiac output using an oesophageal Doppler probe. (1) Measurement of the internal diameter of the ascending aorta; (2) Placement of oesophageal probe; (3) Comparison of oesophageal probe measurement with cardiac output calculated from aortic root diameter and aortic flow velocity measured by a probe in the suprasternal notch.
[3]*and Mark JB, Stenbrook RA et al., Continuous non-invasive monitoring of cardiac output with esophageal Doppler ultrasound during cardiac surgery,* Anesth Analg *1986; 65: 1013–20.*

by means of phased array techniques has enhanced the usefulness of later instruments.[31] Indeed, for monitoring purposes, changes in velocity can be appreciated in a useful manner and converted into an approximation of cardiac output,[30] while the ability of the ultrasound beam to define the edge of dense structures has led to the development of automatic border detection (ABD),[32] yielding visual information on the activity of the heart and its chambers. A succinct account of the transducers, the images (M-mode and B-mode) which they produce, and the construction of the probes is given by Durkin.[33] Other descriptions of probes, including recent developments, are given by Fan *et al*[34] who make comparisons of current instruments, noting that the lack of standardisation in the field is a significant handicap, and by others.[35,36] A more detailed account of the technique and its general applications is that of Clements and Bruijn,[37] whilst others have commented on particular aspects.[38–41] and Orihashi has documented the usefulness of TEE in guiding pulmonary artery catheters into position.[42]

As in transthoracic and suprasternal notch measurements, positioning of the transducer is important, and it is necessary to be able to estimate the diameter of the aorta. Mark used PD to estimate the diameter of the aorta and, at the same time (since the subjects were undergoing cardiac surgery), obtained direct measurements of the aorta through the open chest.[30] Correlation of aortic sizing was poor. The oesophageal probe was

170

arranged to use CWD to produce a record of velocity in the descending aorta. Suprasternal CWD was also used to confirm the velocity and hence the flow through the ascending aorta. This enabled stroke volume to be displayed and cardiac output to be computed from every 12 beats of the heart. Correlation with cardiac output was not considered sufficiently good, although reproducibility was satisfactory and the results acceptable as trend indicators.

A further application, though not strictly monitoring, was derived from the ability of the transoesophageal ultrasound probe to detect atrial thrombi and valvular vegetations and to aid assessments of prosthetic valve function. This led to recognition of wall thickening and subsequently myocardial ischaemia.[43] Indeed, TEE has become accepted as perhaps the most effective method of detecting intraoperative myocardial ischaemia. It appears to be an earlier and better detector than ECG changes.[44] Moreover, wall changes demonstrated by TEE are more common than those revealed by the ECG, including the 12-lead ECG.[45,46] Mangano also claims that TEE can predict perioperative cardiac morbidity, even when unaccompanied by ECG changes, although it must be observed that most of the studies were carried out during cardiac surgery.[43]

The use of TEE as a predictor of morbidity on the basis of intraoperative detection of myocardial ischaemia has also been reported by Eisenberg et al., who also compared the results of applying the technique in non-cardiac surgery with those obtained with the 12-lead ECG and the 2-lead ECG, and with the information gleaned by preoperative clinical examination.[47] Some patients detected by TEE were missed by the other methods, but conversely TEE missed some of those patients already identified by the alternative methods. They concluded that there was little to choose between the approaches. They also noted that better indications were obtained during cardiac surgery, but believed that the rate of improvement in the ultrasound apparatus might soon yield equally valuable data in non-cardiac surgery.

Method

The approach is similar to that used for gastroscopy although in this case the probe carries no optics and is relatively less vulnerable to damage. Local anaesthesia, by local spraying with or without sedation, is usually sufficient. However, since the principle monitoring application is to estimate cardiac output or ventricular ejection during intensive care or general anaesthesia, the degree of sedation or its absence will in all likelihood be dictated by the overall current management policy for the patient in intensive care or by its use during anaesthesia and surgery.

Value of TEE

Opinion on the efficacy of cardiac output monitoring by TEE is divided.[48] The most useful measurements are made when care is taken in positioning the ultrasound probe and the patient remains undisturbed during the measurement. Indeed, during surgical procedures it may prove difficult to maintain a satisfactory probe position.[49] Therefore, although experts in clinical ultrasound have for some time been able to assess abnormalities of the atria, ventricles, and valves of the heart in the adequate surroundings of the cardiology suite, such studies have until recently been generally beyond the scope of those working in the operating theatre and intensive care unit. A recent review of the place of TEE in the practice of anaesthesia by Perrino *et al.* comments on the advent of ABD and the fact that the technique has so far been limited by the lack of a means of obtaining real-time, quantitative data on left ventricular areas and the degree of change taking place, ie, the change in fractional area.[50] They are optimistic that recent developments do enable serial changes in these variables to be followed during surgery. However, the potential consequences of applying or altering therapy on the basis of inadequate ultrasound information are sufficiently serious to have moved some authorities to suggest that only trained operators should be permitted to use the equipment.[48]

Monitoring applications of TEE

Rafferty and Lippmann have described a five-step sequential approach to monitoring using a straightforward technique designed to obtain reliable results routine under the conditions generally prevailing in the operating room and the intensive care unit.[51]

Anaesthesia and intensive care

Cardiac output determination

A number of studies indicate the usefulness of the method during anaesthesia and surgery[30,52,53] and recently good intraoperative correlation between TEE and thermodilution cardiac output estimation has been claimed.[54] Studies in the intensive care setting suggest that TEE is worthy of consideration as a non-invasive alternative to other methods of cardiac output determination.[55-57] However, in some patients movement artefact may mar the estimations and ventilation, with or without PEEP, may produce problems.[58,59]

172

Chamber size

TEE enables the size of the chambers of the heart to be estimated. More important during clinical monitoring, processing of the resultant data can produce images commensurate with changes in the areas of the ventricles, although the displays must be viewed with a certain amount of caution.[60] They have been used as a basis for estimating the degree of preload hypovolaemia in patients.[60-63]

Myocardial contractility

Techniques have been developed for TEE that enable measurement of the elastance of the ventricle,[64] whose volume is calculated echocardiographically. From this, contractility of the muscle may be derived, as may afterload. End-systolic pressure conditions may also be used to derive contractility.[65] Attractive though these approaches may be, they are still new and relatively untested in clinical practice. The use of TEE in assessment of left ventricular function during apnoea in patients thought to have sustained brain-stem damage and who could be candidates for organ donation has been suggested.[66]

Ejection fraction

The popularity of this variable has attracted much attention to non-invasive ways of measuring it. TEE is admirably suited to gauging the shortening of the papillae, a function intimately related to the change in size of the ventricle between systole and diastole or, more strictly, end-systole and end-diastole. The method has been validated.[67]

Wall motion

Atkov *et al.* found TEE was useful for the detection of myocardial ischaemia in more than 70% of patients and noted that only apical ischaemia was missed.[68] Although there is evidence that wall motion detection can be validated, there may be reason once again to exercise some restraint until more clinical experience has been gained.[69]

Air embolism

TEE is established as an effective method of detecting air embolism during neurosurgery and other procedures, such as liver transplantation, in which it may arise.

Complications

The use of TEE seems to be generally free of complications. However, oropharyngeal injury following insertion of the probe, bradycardia thought to be due to the presence of the probe in the oesophagus, buckling of the probe, and difficulty in removing it are among complications reported.[70–73]

In the intensive care setting, the frequency of bacteraemia associated with TEE has been investigated.[74] The use of disposable latex sheaths, instead of repeatedly sterilising these expensive and often delicate instruments, has been recommended.[75]

Impact on decision-making in intensive care

Chenzbraun *et al.* claim that TEE is easily performed in the intensive care unit and that, in their experience, it yields useful information in almost half the cases.[76] They note that it had little success in influencing the management of septicaemic patients, however. Schuster nevertheless found TEE particularly helpful in the evaluation of cardiac size and function in shock, especially in respect of estimating preload in patients receiving inotropes and pressor vasotherapy, but noted that interpretation of measurements was difficult when PEEP was applied.[59] Khoury *et al.* found that TEE was feasible in all the patients in their study, 47% of whom were ventilated.[61] They found that changes in therapy had been prompted by the results obtained from TEE in 60% of the patients, in 48% of whom the change was dictated solely by TEE findings. Lambertz *et al.*, mindful of the appreciable discomfort suffered by some patients during routine TEE, an important consideration in the intensive care unit, make suggestions on how to overcome it.[77]

Emergencies

Several studies have relevance to the management of emergencies. Topics covered include the use of TEE in the diagnosis of intrathoracic bleeding and internal injuries after blunt chest injuries, gunshot wounds of the chest, and the detection of paradoxical gas embolism giving rise to unexpected neurological complications.[78–81]

Measurement of flow in unobstructed blood vessels

Besides qualitative estimation of blood flow, quantitative measurements are now possible. Data obtained continuously from a probe placed over a blood vessel may be processed by microprocessor based computation equipment to produce outputs in both numerical and graphical form, while vascular surgeons find the amplified sound signal based on the reflected ultrasound waves of value in appreciating the pattern of the flow.

Measurement of flow in diseased blood vessels

This is of special value when the probe is moved along a blood vessel. Irregularities of flow at sites of minor occlusion and interference with flow may be located, as may sites of gross occlusion or obliteration. Several specific conditions are worthy of comment.

Arterial

Abnormal arterial configurations are:

Aneurysms

The sites of aneurysms may be determined by ultrasound probe. For example, the distinction between femoral hernia and a saphena varix is an important one.

Fistulae

Similarly, abnormal communications between vessels may be detected. The ultrasound probe may also be valuable in locating implanted vascular shunts.

Abnormal venous configuration

Pathological conditions in veins

It was thought that the deep perforating communications of varicose vein systems might be susceptible to delineation by ultrasound probing, but the technique was found wanting and has been supplanted by alternative approaches.

Thrombosis

The ultrasound probe has been used for the detection of deep vein thrombosis since the introduction of the technique and is still a useful method outside specialist vein clinics. Thus portable hand-held probes

175

are used for post-operative scanning of veins to exclude gross thrombus formation and some clinicians in critical care practice use them for the same reason in patients who are immobile for protracted periods.

Diagnostic scope and limitations

Medical

Surgical practice

Ultrasound is now in widespread use in non-invasive scanning in general surgery, surgical sub-specialities, and obstetrics. Its use in surgical monitoring is more restricted, but has found extensive application in the practice of vascular surgery, both as a surveillance monitoring technique before and after surgery and as an aid in establishing the patency of blood vessels and vascular prostheses and the effectiveness of distal perfusion during the performance of vascular surgical procedures.

Venous occlusion and thrombosis

Similarly, Doppler probes have been used in the detection of thrombosis of the deep veins for many years. Practitioners vary in their enthusiasm for surveillance outside the immediate post-surgical ward and the follow-up clinic, but it might be argued that more extensive use in the period in which post-operative surgical patients are most vulnerable to deep venous thrombosis and embolisation could confer additional benefit.

Use after arterial reconstructive surgery

Post-operative vascular surveillance is important after both major vascular reconstructive surgery and after peripheral vascular procedures. In such circumstances, the equipment should be chosen with care and advice obtained from those with experience in the field. Imaging specialists will often be in the best position to advise on surveillance methods and obtain the best results.

Medical practice

Echocardiography has become a highly developed subset of cardiological investigation. While it behoves clinicians to be familiar with the principles and the potential results to be obtained, expert cardiological opinion should be sought when the performance of chambers of the heart, the heart valves,

176

and the flow through them, and the performance of prosthetic valves need to be monitored.

Stress monitoring

TEE has been employed with success in stress monitoring of suspected cardiac disease.[82,83] Like all cardiac stress monitoring, it is not without risk and the importance of skilled nursing assistance has been emphasised.[84]

Anaesthesia

The use of the transoesophageal ultrasound echocardiographic probe is one the most exciting developments in anaesthetic practice in recent years. Although the absolute accuracy of measurements using the probe may be questioned, the value of the approach lies in the ability to detect abrupt changes or important trends, such as those due to emboli, incipient myocardial ischaemia and serious acute structural and functional cardiac abnormalities.

It is essential that users be versed in the capabilities and limitations of their apparatus in these circumstances, especially as information may be obtained requiring careful assessment in the overall context of anaesthesia, and yet may demand a prompt response.

It is difficult to escape the conclusion that the combined benefits and potential hazards of the technique predicate the establishment of formal programmes of instruction in the theory and practical use of the instruments (see below).

Emergencies

Use in the emergency department

Much of what has been said about the use of ultrasound monitoring using the hand-held devices commonly available for suspected deep vein thrombosis and vascular embolism applies also to the emergency department. It is, however, unlikely that at present mobile monitoring of cardiac function by transthoracic or transoesophageal echocardiography will supplant the need to submit the patient with severe cardiac disease to the expert attentions of the cardiological investigation unit or the well equipped coronary care unit.

Critical care: venous and arterial occlusion

It is doubtful whether the benefits of deep vein monitoring and surveillance in the intensive care unit are being fully realised at present. Routine scanning by hand-held devices is a simple manoeuvre which consumes only a few minutes.

Aortic velography

As has been pointed out, estimation of cardiac output and derived information can be obtained by means of suprasternal notch echocardiography. However, the limitations of the single probe should be appreciated. Arguments have been made in favour of the approach in support of trend indication but, in the absence of correlative results by alternative methods such as thermal dilution cardiac output determination or the use of probes in alternative sites, validity of the instant results must remain doubtful in many instances. Ease of access is an advantage of this non-invasive approach, but the comparable results achieved by transoesophageal echocardiography in experienced hands merits serious consideration. Correct positioning, the avoidance of movement artefact and obtaining information of the type and quality required are increasingly promoted by the computational and imaging features of the latest equipment.[85] Once again, however, it must be urged that monitoring of this kind should not be introduced without the advice of expert practitioners in this kind of imaging and that the experience of other similar critical care units be sought.

Nursing

It has been argued persuasively that nurses with some training can obtain usable results with echocardiography, although the nurses in question worked in environments in which there was close cooperation between medical and nursing staff intimately concerned with particular kinds of patients and illnesses.[7] Their role was not dissimilar to that of nurses involved in ECG monitoring, who assist in the conduct of the monitoring, but become involved in interpretation or response only when they have special responsibilities in the area where the monitoring is being conducted, for example, the CCU or ICU. With the sphere of influence of nursing expanding, the emergence of nurse practitioners with clearly defined areas of responsibility and authority could prompt their greater involvement.

178

General practice

The devolution of more of the care previously the preserve of hospitals to the general practitioner includes the earlier discharge of post-operative patients. As family practitioners undertake more surveillance of these patients, the use of ultrasound in their practices in the detection of postoperative thrombotic complications may be expected to increase.

Need for training and experience

Ultrasound monitoring equipment varies in complexity from the simple hand-held vein scanners to advanced cardiac imaging units. Automation may simplify many tasks and make others reliable in the hands of the relatively untrained. In many instances, interpretation of data requires skill, training, and experience. Past experience indicates that the use of the simpler Doppler devices for the detection of deep vein thrombosis or the follow-up of vascular surgical patients may be well within the competence of general practitioners and nurse practitioners with the benefit of a brief grounding in the basic theory and practical use of the equipment. The instrumentation for the assessment of cardiac performance, however, requires special knowledge and skill on the part of the operator. Transoesophageal monitoring, in particular, because of its apparent simplicity and the ease of obtaining almost instant data, is instantly attractive and can easily, but mistakenly, be regarded as just another exciting new gadget. This is a matter for concern.[86]

Training programmes have been devised,[87-91] but opinions differ on their duration and content,[92,93] and the experience required.[87,94-98] However, many imaging departments have drawn up guidelines for the use of ultrasound imaging equipment and individual training programmes should be pursued in conjunction with imaging departments.

Care of the equipment

Hand-held scanning devices of the simpler type may simply be maintained by the user, perhaps in conjunction with a medical engineering or equivalent facility, in accordance with the manufacturer's instructions.

More complex equipment is likely to contain computational equipment requiring periodic updating or maintenance, while calibration may need to be carried out by authorised personnel on a regular and perhaps frequent basis.[99,100] Quality control is of the greatest importance and should be exercised as part of a formal quality control system, preferably in conjunction with a department of imaging, physics or medical engineering.

179

1 Waggoner AD. Principles and physics of Doppler. *Cardiol Clin* 1990; **8**: 173–90.
2 Huntsman LL, Gams E, Johnson CC, Fairbanks E. Transcutaneous determination of aortic blood-flow velocities in man. *Amer Heart J* 1975; **89**: 605–12.
3 Voyles WF, Greene ER, Miranda IP, Reilly PA. Observer variability in serial noninvasive measurements of stroke index using pulsed Doppler flowmetry. *Biomed Sci Int* 1982; **18**: 67–75.
4 Light LH. Initial evaluation of transcutaneous aortovelography – a new non-invasive technique for hemodynamic measurements in the major thoracic vessels. In *Cardiovascular Applications of Ultrasound*, Reneman RS ed. New York: Elsevier 1974: 325–60.
5 Angelsen BAJ, Brubakk AO. Transcutaneous measurement of blood flow velocity in the human aorta. *Cardiovasc Res* 1976; **10**: 368–79.
6 Gisvold SE, Brubakk AO. Measurement of instantaneous blood-velocity in the human aorta using pulsed Doppler ultrasound. *Cardiovasc Res* 1982; **16**: 26–33.
7 Huntsman LL, Stewart DK, Barnes SR, Franklin SB, Colocousis JS, Hessel EA. Noninvasive Doppler determination of cardiac output in man. Clinical validation. *Circulation* 1983; **67**: 593–602.
8 Clark C, Schulz DL. Velocity distribution in aortic flow. *Cardiovasc Res* 1973; **7**: 601–13.
9 Ihlen H, Amlie JP, Dale J, Forfang K, Nitter-Hauge S, Otterstad JE, *et al*. Determination of cardiac output by Doppler echocardiography. *Br Heart J* 1984; **51**: 54–60.
10 Wells PNT. *Biomedical ultrasonics*. London: Academic Press, 1969, 370–2.
11 Donovan KD, Dobb GJ, Newman MA, Hockings BES, Ireland M. Comparison of pulsed Doppler and thermodilution methods for measuring cardiac output in critically ill patients. *Crit Care Med* 1987; **15**: 853–7.
12 Dobb GJ, Donovan KD. Measuring cardiac output. *Intens Care Med* 1987; **13**: 304–9.
13 Francis GS, Hagan AD, Oury J, O'Rourke RA. Accuracy of echocardiography for assessing aortic root diameter. *Brit Heart J* 1975; **37**: 376–8.
14 Labovitz AJ, Buckingham TA, Habermehl K, Nelson J, Kennedy HL, Williams GA. The effects of sampling site on the two-dimensional echo-Doppler determination of cardiac output. *Amer Heart J* 1985; **109**: 327–32.
15 Merillon JP, Motte G, Fruchaud J, Masquet C, Gourgon R. Evaluation of the elasticity and characteristic impedance of the ascending aorta in man. *Cardiovasc Res* 1978; **12**: 401–6.
16 Levett JM, Replogle RL. Thermodilution cardiac output: a critical analysis and review of the literature. *J Surg Res* 1979; **27**: 392–404.
17 Versprille A. Thermodilution in mechanically ventilated patients. *Intens Care Med* 1984; **10**: 213–5.
18 Sprung CL, Drescher M, Schein RMH. Clinical investigation of the cardiovascular system in the critically ill. Invasive techniques. *Crit Care Clin* 1985; **1**: 533–46.
19 Lang-Jensen T, Berning J, Jacobsen E. Stroke volume measured by pulsed ultrasound Doppler and M-Mode echocardiography. *Acta Anaesthesiol Scand* 1983; **27**: 454–7.
20 Loeppky JA, Hoekanga, Greene ER, Luft UC. Comparison of noninvasive pulsed Doppler and Fick measurements of stroke volume in cardiac patients. *Am Heart J* 1984; **107**: 339–46.
21 Nishimura RA, Callahan MJ, Schaff HV, Ilstrup DM, Miller FA, Tajik AJ. Noninvasive measurement of cardiac output by continuous-wave Doppler echocardiography: initial experience and review of the literature. *Mayo Clin Proc* 1984; **59**: 484–9.
22 Ihlen H, Muhre E, Amlie JP, Forfang K, Larsen S. Changes in left ventricular stroke volume measured by Doppler echocardiography. *Br Heart J* 1985; **54**: 378–83.
23 Gardin JM, Burn C, Hughes C, Henry WL. Are Doppler aortic flow velocity measurements reproducible? *Circulation* (abstr) 1981; **64** (suppl IV): IV–205.
24 Gisvold SE, Brubakk AO: Measurement of instantaneous blood-velocity in the human aorta using pulsed Doppler ultrasound. *Cardiovasc Res* 1982; **16**: 26–33.
25 Hoenecke HR, Goldberg SJ, Carnahan Y, Sahn DJ, Allen HD, Valdes-Cruz LM. Controlled quantitative assessment of pulmonary and aortic flow by range gated pulsed Doppler in children with cardiac disease. *Circulation* (abst) 1981; **64** (suppl IV): IV–167.
26 Elkayam U, Gardin JM, Berkley R, Hughes CA, Henry WL. The use of Doppler flow velocity measurements to assess the hemodynamic response to vasodilation in patients with heart failure. *Circulation* 1983; **67**: 377–83.

27 Rein AJJ, Hsieh KS, Elixon M, Colan SD, Lang P, Sanders SP, *et al*. Cardiac output estimates in the pediatric intensive care unit using a continuous-wave Doppler computer: Validation and limitations of the technique. *Am Heart J* 1986; **112**: 97–103.

28 Alverson DC, Eldridge M, Dillon T, Yabek SM, Berman W. Noninvasive pulsed Doppler determination of cardiac output in neonates and children. *J Pediatr* 1982; **101**: 46–50.

29 Mellander M, Sabel K-G, Caidahl K, Solymar L, Eriksson B. Doppler determination of cardiac output in infants and children: Comparison with thermodilution. *Pediatr Cardiol* 1987; **8**: 241–6.

30 Mark JB, Steinbrook RA, Gugino LD, Maddi R, Hartwell B, Shemin R, *et al*. Continuous non-invasive monitoring of cardiac output with esophageal Doppler ultrasound during cardiac surgery. *Anesth Analg* 1986; **65**: 1013–20.

31 Schluter M, Langenstein BA, Polster J, Kremer P, Souquet J, Engel S, *et al*. Transoesophageal cross-sectional echocardiography with a phased array transducer system: technique and initial clinical results. *Brit Heart J* 1982; **48**: 67–72.

32 Katz WE, Gasior TA, Reddy SC, Goresan J 3rd. Utility and limitations of biplane transesophageal echocardiographic automated border detection for estimation of left ventricular stroke volume and output. *Amer Heart J* 1994; **128**: 389–96.

33 Durkin M. Echocardiography. In: Hutton P, Prys-Roberts C, eds. *Monitoring in anaesthesia and intensive care*. London: WB Saunders Company Ltd, 1994.

34 Fan PH, Anayiotos A, Nanda NC, Yoganathan AP, Cape EG. Intramachine variability in transesophageal color Doppler images of pulsatile jets. In vitro studies. *Circulation* 1994; **89**: 2141–9.

35 Djoa KK, Lance CT, De Jong N, Linker DT, Bom N. Transesophageal transducer technology: an overview. *Amer J Cardiol Imaging* 1995; **9**: 79–86.

36 Waltman TJ, Dittrich HC. What's new in transesophageal echocardiography? *Curr Opin Cardiol* 1994; **9**: 709–20.

37 Clements FM, Bruijin NP. *Transesophageal echocardiography*. Boston: Little Brown, 1991.

38 Roewer N, Greim CA. Perioperative applications of transesophageal echocardiography. *Anasthesiol Intensivmed Notfallmed Schmerzther* 1994; **29**: 458–74.

39 Goertz A, Georgieff M. Intraoperative transesophageal echocardiography – possibilities and prospects. *Anasthesiol Intensivmed Notfallmed Schmerzther* 1994; **29**: 456–7.

40 Martin RP. Real time ultrasound quantification of ventricular function: has the eyeball been replaced or will the subjective become objective? *J Amer Coll Cardiol* 1992; **19**: 321–3.

41 Seward JB, Khanderia BK, Oh JK, Freeman WK. Critical appraisal of transesophageal echocardiography: limitations, pitfalls, and complications. *J Amer Soc Echocardiogr* 1992; **5**: 288–305.

42 Orihashi K, Nakashima Y, Sueda T, Yuge O, Matsuura Y. Usefulness of transesophageal echocardiography for guiding pulmonary artery catheter placement in the operating room. *Heart Vessels* 1994: **9**: 315–21.

43 Mangano DT. Perioperative cardiac morbidity. *Anesthesiology* 1990; **72**: 153–84.

44 Wohlgelernter D, Cleman M, Highman HA, Fetterman RC, Duncan JS, Zaret BL, *et al*. Regional myocardial dysfunction during coronary angioplasty: evaluation by two-dimensional echocardiography and 12-lead electrocardiography. *J Amer Coll Cardiol* 1986; **7**: 1245–54.

45 Smith MD, Macphail B, Harrison ME, Lenhoff SJ, De Maria AN. Value and limitations of transesophageal echocardiography in determination of left ventricular volumes and ejection fraction. *J Amer J Coll Cardiol* 1992; **19**: 1213–22.

46 Leung JM, Levine EH. Left ventricular end-systolic cavity obliteration as an estimate of intraoperative hypovolemia. *Anesthesiology* 1994; **81**: 1102–9.

47 Eisenberg MJ, London MJ, Leung JM, Browner WS, Hollenberg M, Tubau JF, *et al*. Monitoring for myocardial ischemia during noncardiac surgery. A technology assessment of transesophageal echocardiography and 12-lead electrocardiography. *JAMA* 1992; **268**: 210–16.

48 Pearlman AS. Transesophageal echocardiography: sound diagnosis or two edged sword? *N Engl J Med* 1991; **324**: 841–3.

49 Perrino AC, Fleming J, LeMantia KR. Transesophageal cardiac output monitoring: performance during aortic reconstructive surgery. *Anesth Analg* 1991; **73**: 705–10.

50 Perrino AC, Luther MA, O'Connor TZ, Cohen IS. Automated echocardiographic analysis. Examination of serial intraoperative measurements. *Anesthesiology* 1995; **83**: 285–92.

51 Rafferty TD, Lippmann H. Intraoperative two-dimensional echocardiography and color flow, Doppler imaging: a basic transesophageal single plane patient examination sequence. *Yale Biol Med* 1993; **66**: 349–83.

52 Kremer P, Cahalan M, Beaupre P, Schroder E, Hanrath P, Heinrich H, *et al.* Intraoperative monitoring using transesophageal 2-dimensional echocardiography. *Anaesthesist* 1985; **34**: 111–7.

53 Schmid ER, Spahn DR, Tornic M. Reliability of a new generation transesophageal Doppler device for cardiac output monitoring. *Anesth Analg* 1993; 77: 971–9.

54 Darmon PL, Hillel Z, Mogtader A, Mindich B, Thys D. Cardiac output by transesophageal echocardiography using continuous-wave Doppler across the aortic valve. *Anesthesiology* 1994; **80**: 796–805.

55 Oh JK, Seward JB, Khanderia BK, Gersh BJ, McGregor CG, Freeman WK, *et al.* Transesophageal echocardiography in critically ill patients. *Amer J Cardiol.* 1990; **66**: 1492–5.

56 Porembka DT, Hoitt BD. Transesophageal echocardiography in the intensive care patient. *Crit Care Med* 1991; **19**: 826–35.

57 Peterson JW, Orsinelli. Transesophageal echocardiography. When is it superior to standard imaging in clinical practice? *Postgrad Med* 1995; **97**: 43–61.

58 Koolen JJ, Visser CA, Wever E, van Wesel H, Meyne NG, Dunning AJ. Transesophageal two-dimensional echocardiographic evaluation of biventricular dimension and function during positive end-expiratory pressure ventilation after coronary bypass grafting. *Amer J Cardiol* 1987; **59**: 1047–51.

59 Schuster S. Transesophageal echocardiography on the intensive care unit. *Herz* 1993; **18**: 361–71.

60 Cheung AT, Savino JS, Weiss SJ, Aukburg SJ, Berlin JA. Echocardiographic and hemodynamic indexes of left ventricular preload in patients with normal and abnormal ventricular function. *Anesthesiology* 1994; **81**: 376–87.

61 Khoury AF, Afridi I, Quinones MA, Zoghbi WA. Transesophageal echocardiography in critically ill patients: feasibility, safety, and impact on management. *Amer Heart J* 1994; **127**: 1363–71.

62 Perez de Prado A, Garcia-Fernandez MA, Barambio M, Moreno M, Torecilla EG, San Roman D, *et al.* The usefulness of transesophageal echocardiography in general intensive care units. *Rev Esp Cardiol* 1994; **47**: 735–40.

63 van Daele ME, Trouwborst A, van Woerkens LC, Tenbrinck R, Fraser AG, Roelandt JR. Transesophageal echocardiographic monitoring of preoperative acute hypervolemic hemodilution. *Anesthesiology* 1994; **81**: 602–9.

64 Hillel Z, Thys DM, Mindich BP, Goldman ME, Kaplan JA. A new method for intraoperative determination of contractility. *Anesth Analg* 1986; **65**: 572.

65 Gorcsan J 3rd, Gasior TA, Mandarino WA, Deneault LG, Hattler BG, Pinsky MR. Assessment of the immediate effects of cardiopulmonary bypass on left ventricular performance by on-line pressure-area relations. *Circulation* 1994; **89**: 180–90.

66 Orliaget GA, Catoire P, Liu N, Beydon L, Bonnet F. Transesophageal echocardiographic assessment of left ventricular function during apnea testing for brain death. *Transplantation* 1994; **58**: 655–8.

67 Doerr HK, Quinones MA, Zoghbi WA. Accurate determination of left ventricular ejection fraction by transesophageal echocardiography with a nonvolumetric method. *J Amer Soc Echocardiogr* 1993; **6**: 476–81.

68 Atkov OYu, Akchurin RS, Tkachuk LM, Lepilin MG, Sukernik MR. Intraoperative transesophageal echocardiography for the detection of myocardial ischemia. *Herz* 1993; **18**: 372–8.

69 Harris SN, Gordon MA, Urban MK, O'Connor TZ, Barash PG. The pressure rate quotient is not an indicator of myocardial ischemia in humans. *Anesthesiology* 1993; **78**: 242–50.

70 Savino JS, Hanson CW 3rd, Bigelow DC, Cheung AT, Weiss SJ. Oropharyngeal injury following transesophageal echocardiography. *J Cardiothorac Vasc Anesth* 1994; **8**: 76–8.

71 Suriani RJ, Tzou N. Bradycardia during transesophageal echocardiographic probe. *J Cardiothorac Vasc Anesth* 1995; **9**: 347.

72 Orihashi K, Sueda T, Matsuura Y, Tamanoue T, Yuge O. Buckling of transesophageal echocardiography probe: a pitfall at insertion in an anesthetized patient. *Hiroshima J Med Sci* 1993; **42**: 155–7.

73 Woodland RV, Denney JD, Moore DW, Gregg MG. Inability to remove a transesophageal echocardiography probe. *J Cardiothorac Vasc Anesth* 1994; **8**: 477–9.

74 Mentec H, Vignon P, Terre S, Cholley B, Roupie E, Legrand P, *et al.* Frequency of bacteraemia associated with transesophageal echocardiography in intensive care unit patients: a prospective study of 139 patients. *Crit Care Med* 1995; **23**: 1194–9.

75 Fritz S, Hust MH, Ochs C, Gratwohl I, Staiger M, Braun B. Use of a latex cover sheath for transesophageal echocardiography (TEE) instead of regular disinfection of the scope. *Clin Cardiol* 1993: **16**: 737–40.

76 Chenzbraun A, Pinto JF, Schnittger I. Transesophageal echocardiography in the intensive care unit: impact on diagnosis and decision-making. *Clin Cardiol* 1994; **17**: 434–44.

77 Lambertz H, Menzel T, Stellwaag M. Comparison of conventional and miniaturized biplane echoscope: initial clinical results. *Z Kardiol* 1994; **83**: 666–71.

78 Le Bret F, Ruel P, Rosier H, Goarin JP, Rouin B, Viars P. Diagnosis of traumatic mediastinal haematoma with transesophageal echocardiography. *Chest* 1994; **105**: 373–6. (Erratum in *Chest* 1994; **105**: 1924.)

79 Karalis DG, Victor MF, Davis GA, McAllister MP, Covalesky VA, Ross JJ Jr *et al.* The role of echocardiography in blunt chest trauma: a transthoracic and transesophageal echcardiographic study. *J Trauma* 1994; **36**: 53–8.

80 McIntyre RC Jr, Moore EE, Read RR, Wiebe RL, Grover FL. Transesophageal echocardiography in the evaluation of a transmediastinal gunshot would: case report. *J Trauma* 1994; **36**: 125–7.

81 Boussuges A, Blanc P, Habib G. Neurologic accident of decompression: a new indication of transesophageal echocardiography. *Presse Médicale* 1995; **24**: 853–4.

82 Panza JA, Laurienzo JM, Curiel RV, Quyyumi AA, Cannon RO 3rd. Transesophageal dobutamine stress echocardiography for evaluation of patients with coronary artery disease. *J Amer Coll Cardiol* 1994; **24**: 1260–7.

83 Kamp O, Visser CA. Improved detection of wall plane motion by transesophageal stress echocardiography using a biplane transducer. *Amer J Cardiol Imaging* 1995; **9**: 137–141.

84 Laurienzo JM. Transesophageal dobutamine stress echcardiography: the nurse's role. *J Cardiovasc Nurs* 1995; **9**: 24–35.

85 Font VE, Obarski TP, Klein AL *et al.* Transesophageal echocardiography in the critical care unit. *Cleve Clin J Med* 1991; **58**: 315–22.

86 Savage DD, Garrison RJ, Kannel WB, Anderson SJ, Feinleib M, Castell WP. Considerations in the use of echocardiography in epidemiology. The Framingham Study. *Hypertension* 1987; **9**: 1140–4.

87 Pearlman AS, Gardin JM, Martin RP, Parisi AF, Popp RL, Quinones MA, *et al.* Guidelines for physician training in transesophageal echocardiography: recommendations of the American Society of Echocardiography Committee for Training in Echocardiography. *J Amer Soc Cardiogr* 1992; **5**: 187–94.

88 Gardner CJ, Brown S, Hagen-Ansert S, Harrigan P, Kisslo J, Kisslo K, *et al.* Guidelines for cardiac sonographer education: report of the American Society of Echocardiography Sonographer Education Committee. *J Amer Soc Echocardiogr* 1992; **5**: 635–9.

89 Roudaut R, Touche T, Cohen A, Cormier B, Dehant P, Diebold B, *et al.* Guidelines of the French Society of Cardiology on the training of echocardiographers and the performing of echocardiography. *Arch Mal Coeur Vaiss* 1994; **87**: 791–8.

90 Meyer RA, Hagler D, Huhta J, Smallham J, Snider R, Williams R. Guidelines for physician training in pediatric echocardiography. *Amer J Cardiol* 1987; **60**: 164–5.

91 Savage RM, Licina MG, Koch CG, Hearn CJ, Thomas JD, Starr NJ, *et al.* Educational program for intraoperative transesophageal echocardiography. *Anesth Analg* 1995; **81**: 399–403.

92 Reves JG, Schell RM. Education for cardiac anesthesia. In: Estafanous FG, Barash PG, Reves JG eds. *Cardiac anesthesia*. Philadelphia: JB Lippincott, 1994.

93 Cahalan MK, Foster E. Training in transesophageal echocardiography: in the lab or on the job? *Anesth Analg* 1995; **81**: 217–8.

94 Picano E, Lattanzi F, Orlandini A. Stress echocardiography and the an factor: the importance of being expert. *J Amer Coll Cardiol* 1991: **17**: 666–9.

95 Ungerleider RM. Greeley WJ, Kanter RJ, Kisslo JA. The learning curve for intraoperative echocardiography during congenital heart surgery. *Ann Thorac Surg* 1992; **54**: 691–6.

96 Foster E, Redberg RF, Schiller NB. Transesophageal echocardiography. Indications and technical considerations. *Cardiol Clin* 1993; **11**: 355–60.

97 Sloth E, Hasenkam JM, Kristensen BO, Jakobsen CJ, Nygaard H, Juhl B. Transesophageal echocardiography for registration of hemodynamics. A new tool in anesthesiology. *Ugeskr Laeger* 1993; **155**: 3989–93.

98 Health Equipment Information No. 98: *Management of medical equipment and devices.* London: Department of Health, 1991.

99 MDA. *The Report of the expert working group on alarms on clinical monitors.* London: Medical Devices Agency, 1995.

100 Rafferty T, Lamantia K, Davis E, Phillips D, Harris S, Carter J, *et al.* Quality assurance for intraoperative transesophageal echocardiography monitoring: a report of 846 procedures. *Anesth Analg* 1993; **76**: 228–32.

Further reading

Taylor KJW, Burns PN, Wells PN, eds. *Clinical applications of Doppler ultrasound.* London: Academic Press, 1988.

Missri J. *Transesophageal echocardiography: clinical and intraoperative applications.* New York: Churchill Livingstone, 1993.

Chambers JB. *Clinical echocardiography.* BMJ Publishing Group, 1995. (A general clinical review.)

Rafferty TD. *Basics of transesophageal echocardiography.* New York: Churchill Livingstone, 1995. (An up-to-date, yet concise, review of the applications of the technique, with an emphasis on anaesthesia and intensive care)

14 Electrical impedance monitoring

Background and physical principles

When a high frequency alternating current is passed through a non-homogeneous body, the impedance encountered is that of the disparate components. Of these, the air breathed is of little importance, but muscle, blood and the other tissues make significant contributions. It may be assumed for convenience that, apart from the blood content of the heart and lungs, the composition and characteristics of the remaining tissues (in terms of impedance) may be regarded as constant. Changes in impedance are therefore capable of being correlated with changes in the blood volume contained in the thorax (see Figure 14.1).

Thoracic impedance monitoring

The technique was introduced into medicine by Nyboer, who applied it to the measurement of flow in limbs,[1] although Atzler and Lehmann had postulated a relationship between transthoracic impedance and events in

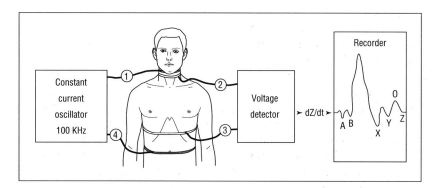

Figure 14.1 Diagrammatic representation of the equipment used to measure thoracic impedance. An oscillator provides a current source which is applied to the neck 1 and trunk 4. Electrodes also placed on the neck 2 and trunk 3 detect an output voltage which, as a signal representing dZ/dt, is amplified and conducted to a recorder or a suitable display device. Redrawn from Donovan GJ and Dobb KD. Non-invasive methods of measuring cardiac output. Intens Care Med. 1989; **13**: 304–9.

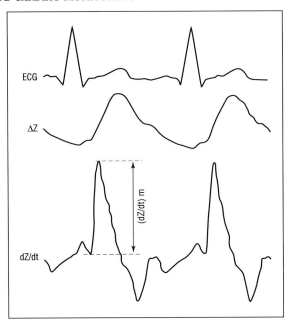

ECG

ΔZ

(dZ/dt) m

dZ/dt

Figure 14.2 ECG and impedance plethysmogram. Z is the trace of changes in thoracic impedance during the cardiac cycle. dZ/dt max is the time derivative of Z and is used in calculating stroke volume. ᴮand BoMed Medical Manufacturing Ltd.

the cardiac cycle in 1932.[2] Since the impedance of the thorax changes according to the amount of blood present,[3-5] it is tempting to postulate that changes in stroke volume of the heart should change the impedance in a predictable fashion.[6]

Three pairs of electrodes are placed circumferentially about the subject.[7] One is fitted around the neck and the other two around the upper abdomen and thorax. The potential difference between what are in effect the inner electrodes and the outer electrodes is sensed when a high frequency alternating current is applied. Since breathing also changes the impedance of the thorax, the method formerly had the drawback of needing to be applied during breath-holding or apnoea, or the effects of breathing needed to be eliminated by detection of the synchronous activity of the heart to the exclusion of the asynchronous breathing pattern. Current instruments use algorithms designed to minimise the effects of respiratory interference to the point where they bear reasonable comparison with their invasive counterparts. Typical output is shown in Figure 14.2.

Although the technique has been available for many years and despite having the advantage of being non-invasive,[8,9] it failed initially to achieve a firm place in the routine measurement of cardiac output.[10] Whereas the early studies were satisfactory,[4] others found the correlation with dye

186

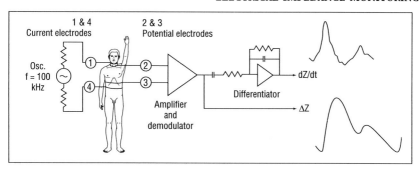

Figure 14.3 Diagrammatic representation of a thoracic bioimpedance measurement system. As indicated, an oscillating current is applied through electrodes 1 and 4 and an output voltage sensed by electrodes 2 and 4. An amplifier takes the output signal and its carrier signal. The output of the amplifier is differentiated as shown to yield dZ/dt. When plotted with respect to time, this yields the trace shown above right and this corresponds to the cardiac output waveform shown below right.[A]

dilution and thermal dilution cardiac output methods disappointing and the technique came to be generally regarded as unreliable in clinical practice. It has been pointed out that the original studies concerned fit young subjects (astronauts), in whom acceptable results were obtained, whereas the results obtained from the sick and elderly, the latter often having a poor posture or frank skeletal deformities, were inferior.[11,12] It appeared that the equation for the calculation of cardiac output, using the first derivative of the electrical impedance, dZ/dt (Z is the symbol for the impedance in ohms), was wanting.[13] Sramek and Bernstein tackled the problem and produced a new equation, now often referred to as the Sramek-Bernstein equation,[14,15] which has been validated for rest and exercise[16] and has been incorporated into the BoMed NCCOM 3 instrument.[11,17] The general arrangement of a thoracic bioimpedance system in shown in Figure 14.3.

Theory of operation

The theory underlying the clinical operation of thoracic bioimpedance measuring instruments but may be summarised, as follows.

The thorax acts as a conducting medium between electrodes placed at the level of the xiphisternum and at the root of the neck. At rest, the thorax thus connected has an electrical impedance which we may call Z_o. The value Z_o ohms is taken as a baseline for measurement and the contents are regarded as homogeneous. Since the various constituents of the thorax contribute to its total impedance, change in any of them should alter the value of Z. In the event, we are interested in changes relating to the flow in the aorta and which are of a pulsatile nature; and, in fact, a trace of the changes in Z corresponding to the pulsatile aortic flow resembles that of

Theory

It can be shown that the maximum rate of change of Z is proportional to the peak flow in the ascending aorta[6] yielding the formula:

$$SV = \frac{\rho L^2 T \left(\dfrac{\delta Z}{\delta t} \right) \text{max}}{Z_0^{\,2}}$$

where SV = stroke volume (ml)
  ρ = resistivity of blood (ohm.cm)
  L = distance between the sensing electrodes
  T = left ventricular ejection time (s)

Z_0 varies with ventilation and, indeed, is used in respiratory impedance monitoring, but the change in impedance due to pulsatile aortic flow is much less susceptible to the influence of ventilation, that is:

$$\left(\frac{\delta Z}{\delta t} \right) \text{max}$$

is relatively immune to the ventilatory effects reflected in the value of Z_0. The resistivity of blood[19] ρ is virtually constant throughout a wide range of haematocrit values in a variety of physiological derangements.[20-22] Sramek made the assumption, for practical purposes, that the thorax was a cylinder whose dimensions between the electrodes were:

$$V_{cyl} = \frac{C^2 L}{4\pi}$$

where C = the circumference of the thoracic cylinder
and L = its length

and, since the units of the term $\rho(L^2/Z_0^2)$ in Kubicek's equation were ml.ohm^{-1}, represented the ratio between Z_0 and the effective thoracic tissue volume (which he designated as V_{eppt}) and, having determined that the proportion of the thoracic cylinder functionally taking part in the electrical impedance was 1/2·8, he revised the equation to the form:

$$V_{eppt} = \frac{C^2 L}{2 \cdot 8 \times 4\pi}$$

Theory (continued)

If account is taken of $\left(\dfrac{\delta Z}{\delta t}\right)$ and Z_0,

the previous equation can be rearranged to:

$$SV = \frac{C^2 LT\left(\dfrac{\delta Z}{\delta t}\right)\text{max}}{2\cdot 8 \times 4\pi}$$

This was then simplified further to the more manageable form:

$$SV = VEPT \times \frac{EVI}{TFI} \times VET$$

where $\quad VEPT = V_{\text{eptt}}$
$\qquad VET = T$
$\qquad EVI = (\delta Z/\delta t)\,\text{max}$
and $\qquad TFI = Z_0$

Sramek, as a result of examining radiographs and taking thoracic measurements, found that the ratio of C to L was, to all intents and purposes, $3\cdot 0$ rather than $2\cdot 8$ for almost all subjects (except neonates, for whom the appropriate value was $2\cdot 6$).

Thus, since $VEPT = \dfrac{L^3}{4\cdot 25}$, then $SV = \dfrac{L^3 \times VET \times EVI}{4\cdot 25 \times TFI}$

the arterial pressure waveform with a timing corresponding to the events of the ECG, with the customary delay (Figure 14.4).[18]

Practical application

This is the basis for a development of the original Kubicek concept as the NCCOM 3 (BoMed Medical Manufacturing, Irvine CA), where the length of the thoracic cylinder (L) is taken from a table based on the patient's weight.

Correlation studies have shown wide variation, usually with displacement of the regression line from the line of identity. The studies have compared the electrical bioimpedance method with cardiac output measurements based on the Fick principle[23] or on dye or thermal dilution

189

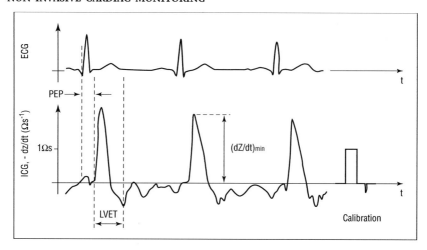

Figure 14.4 ECG and impedance plethysmogram. [A]*and Bleicher W 1982. Possibilities and limitations of thoracic impedance cardiography.* [A,C]*Cardiovascular Measurement in Anaesthesiology. European Academy of Anaesthesiology Proceedings, Berlin, Springer-Verlag (1981) 212–34.*

techniques,[9,23,24] and with Doppler echocardiography.[25] Some have claimed good correlation with Fick[26] and dye dilution methods,[8,27,28] whereas others have considered correlation with other methods poor.[9,14,29] Observer bias may be incurred by the less experienced applying the technique.[30]

It has been pointed out that the instruments have nevertheless been getting better and may be expected to be improved still further,[29] but authors of recent comparative studies still have reservations about the method.[31–33]

The absolute values obtained may depend on the type of electrodes used, whereas the validity of trends and rates of change seems unaffected.[34–36] Some believe that the method may still not be sufficiently validated for satisfactory clinical use,[37,38] and it is noted that it is unsatisfactory in patients with cardiomyopathy and valvular regurgitation, and in those with cardiovascular distortion following cardiac surgery.[39–41]

Certain areas have received special attention. The use of thoracic bioimpedance techniques in stress and exercise testing has been reported on favourably.[42–44] It is considered satisfactory in the estimation of stroke volume as compared with other conventional methods, especially in the elderly,[45] but unsuitable for estimation of the ejection fraction, where it is recommended that it should not be used when radionucleide ventriculography is available.[46] A certain amount of interest has been generated by its possible use in the estimation of lung water and, hence, pulmonary oedema, but this does not appear to have led to effective clinical exploitation.[47–49] Transthoracic bioimpedance has been used with apparent

190

success in trials of drugs with cardiovascular effects and has been recommended as suitable for military use.[50–52]

Intraoperative use

Transthoracic bioimpedance seems to give results similar to those obtained from conventional methods of assessing cardiac output and valuable trend indication intraoperatively.[53]

Intensive care

Studies have been conducted to establish whether or not this attractive, non-invasive method can be regarded as an acceptable alternative to conventional invasive methods of estimating cardiac output and other important cardiovascular variables in adults, children, infants and neonates.[54–60] Again, the estimation of stroke volume has been reported on favourably.[61]

The usefulness of the instrument in the intensive care of patients with septicaemia was examined by Young and McQuillan,[62] who concluded that correlation between dye dilution estimations and those obtained with the BoMed instrument were poor and that the results could not be relied upon in this group of patients, confirming the impression gleaned in an earlier study of post-cardiac bypass patients (Figure 14.5).[63]

Paediatrics

O'Connell et al. have suggested corrections for use of the device in children.[18] They compared cardiac output estimations produced by the instrument with those obtained by dye dilution and found reasonable correlation, as did Mickell et al.[60] However, they noted that measurements of the thoracic cylinder as presented by real patients were critical to satisfactory results. Views differ on the influence exerted by positive end-expiratory pressure (PEEP) in these circumstances.[38,64]

The promise of the technique still remains to be wholly fulfilled, although the BoMed instrument has been progressively improved and a multi-centre study of the use of transthoracic bioimpedance in the intensive care setting should encourage such improvement and prompt continued investigation into the applicability of the technique in the critically ill.[65]

191

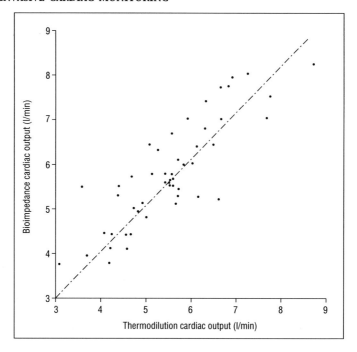

Figure 14.5 Relationship between the impedance cardiogram and thoracic impedance. Traces of the impedance cardiogram (ICG) derived from dZ/dt and of thoracic impedance (Z) taken from a normal subject are shown, together with the temporal relationships between these traces and left ventricular ejection time (LVET) and the pre-ejection period (LVET). The electrocardiogram (ECG) is shown for comparison. Redrawn from Bleicher W 1982. Prys-Roberts C and Vickers MD, eds. Cardiovascular Measurement in Anaesthesiology. European Academy of Anaesthesiology Proceedings, Berlin, Springer-Verlag (1981) 212–34.

Clinical use

Electrode application

The sites chosen for electrode application are intended to encompass the thoracic volume. Pairs of electrodes are therefore applied to the lower thorax and upper abdomen and to the neck.

Good contact and fixing are essential, but difficult to maintain. Other sources of impedance, especially changing impedance, must be minimised. Because of these problems oesophageal siting has been suggested.[66]

General medical and surgical practice

From time to time attempts have been made to introduce electrical impedance monitoring into general medical and surgical practice. There

192

seems to be no reason in theory why the method should not be successful. However, the difficulties of siting the electrodes ideally and maintaining good contact and the need for skilled supervision may be the reason why it has not been widely adopted.

Obstetrics

Patients requiring close and dedicated care, as in pre-eclampsia and in certain post-natal conditions, have been monitored by electrical impedance.[67] The results have been satisfactory and it appears that there is scope for the method under these circumstances.

Neonatal and paediatric medicine

Some success has been reported in neonates, infants and children.[18,60] Again, it seems likely that the presence of dedicated staff contributes to this success, whilst the stillness of some of these small patients is an advantage.

Critical care

The reasons for the poorer correlation between thoracic bioimpedance cardiac output measurements and those obtained from other popular methods have not been established. However, compared with the thermal dilution method bioimpedance generally overestimates low cardiac outputs and underestimates high cardiac outputs.[61,63] Excessive shunting of blood through skin and muscle vessels has been suggested as one possible cause of error.[14] It has also been suggested that certain errors may be attributed to sepsis.[68] Nevertheless, although absolute values should be disregarded, it is possible to obtain useful trend indication. Other reported limitations include reduction in bioimpedance in the presence of pleural effusion or other fluid collections or pulmonary oedema and increases in bioimpedance when a pneumothorax was present or the patient was suffering from obstructive pulmonary disease or was dehydrated.[69,70] Perhaps the contents of the thorax should not be regarded as homogeneous. After all, the impedance decreases during systole and increases during diastole. In terms of changes in pulmonary blood volume, this would seem to be paradoxical in the homogeneous example.[62]

Diagnostic scope and limitations

The advantages and disadvantages are shown in the accompanying box.

Advantages and disadvantages of electrical impedance monitoring

Aggregation of effects

- Since all changes in blood volume are lumped together, high output states in which there is excess blood in the zone of detection of the monitoring electrodes offset the changes genuinely due to stroke volume, so that the stroke volume is likely to be underestimated.
- In conditions in which there is appreciable bi-directional flow, such as aortic regurgitation, underestimates may occur.

Clinical usefulness

- Estimation of cardiac output by the bioimpedance method shows good correlation in the laboratory and has been claimed to yield acceptable results in diagnostic clinics.
- Nevertheless, it does require stable conditions such as are not available in some forms of treatment (eg, intensive care) and users need to be thoroughly familiar with the method to exploit it successfully.

A clinical pitfall

Changes in posture and rapid changes in blood volume may be important during thoracic impedance monitoring.

- There is an appreciable change (of the order of 400 ml) between the upright and supine postures and vice versa.
- Rapid transfusion, eg, in the case of hypovolaemic patients, changes intrapulmonary blood volume.
- Although the algorithms used by thoracic impedance instruments cater for gradual changes, the effects of more rapid changes must be borne in mind and frequent recalibration may be needed.

Safety

- Provided electrically safe equipment complying with the appropriate General and Particular Standards[71-72] for the safety of medical electrical equipment is used, and users are conversant with the potential electrical hazards of electrical equipment connected to patients,[73] the technique appears to be virtually free of hazard.[18]

Interpretation

From the foregoing, it will be evident that there are a number of details of technique to be considered when opting for thoracic impedance monitoring, such that their neglect may lead to error if the results are taken at face value. It is likely that, in many cases, no parallel cardiovascular monitoring is being conducted which will help in assessment of the validity of the results obtained. At the same time, the signals obtained can be displayed as a waveform which closely resembles the pulse waveform. If such provision is made, the user should take care to determine whether the amplitude of the displayed waveform, if it appears to be of normal contour and amplitude, is indeed normal and has not been amplified to yield an easily appreciated trace. The situation is analogous to that of the "normalised" pulse oximetry trace used primarily to demonstrate that the pulse oximeter probe has been applied correctly and the readings thereby validated to that extent. Amplification may have been applied for this purpose only and have no true correlation with the adequacy of the circulation. As with other techniques not yet widely used, it may take some time for those invoking it in monitoring to become aware of its foibles, advantages, and drawbacks in the same way that they have acquired intimate knowledge and experience of more familiar techniques. It should probably not be used as a first line monitoring technique by those who have not already acquired some experience of it.

1 Nyboer J. *Electrical Impedance Plethysmography*. Springfield, Illinois: CC Thomas Co, 1959.
2 Geddes LA, Baker LE. *Principles of Applied Biomedical Instrumentation*, 2nd ed. New York: John Wiley and Sons, 1975: 276–410.
3 Bonjor FH, van den Berg JW, Dirken MN. The origin of the variations in body impedance occurring during the cardiac cycle. *Circulation* 1952; **6**: 415–20.
4 Kubicek WG, Karnegis JN, Patterson RP, Witsoe DA, Mattson RH. Development and evaluation of an impedance cardiac output system. *Aerospace Med* 1966; **37**: 1208–12.
5 Hill DW, Thompson FD. The importance of blood resistivity in the measurement of cardiac output by by the thoracic impedance method. *Med Biol Eng Comput* 1975; **13**: 187–91.
6 Karnegis JN, Heinz J, Kubicek WG. The effect of atrial rhythm on the thoracic impedance cardiogram. *Amer J Med Sci* 1980; **280**: 17–20.
7 Kubicek WG, Kottke FJ, Ramos MU, Patterson RP, Witsoe DA, Labree JW, *et al*. The Minnesota impedance cardiograph – theory and applications. *Biomed Eng* 1974; **9**: 410–6.
8 Dobb GJ, Donovan KD. Non-invasive methods of measuring cardiac output. *Intens Care Med* 1987; **13**: 304–9.
9 Porter JM, Swain ID. Measurement of cardiac output by electrical impedance plethysmography. *J Biomed Eng* 1987; **9**: 222–31.
10 Tremper KK. Continuous non-invasive output: are we getting there? *Crit Care Med* 1987; **15**: 278–9.
11 Appel PL, Kram HB, MacKabee J, Fleming AW, Shoemaker WC. Comparison of measurements of cardiac output by bioimpedance and thermodilution in severely ill surgical patients. *Crit Care Med* 1986; **14**: 933–5.
12 Keim HJ, Wallace JM, Thurston H, Case DB, Drayer JIM, Laragh JH. Impedance cardiography for determination of stroke index. *J Appl Physiol* 1976; **41**: 797–9.

13 Kobayashi Y, Andoh Y, Fujinami T, Nakayama K, Takada K, Takeuchi T, *et al.* Impedance cardiography for estimating cardiac output during submaximal and maximal work. *J Appl Physiol* 1978; **45**: 459–62.

14 Bernstein DP. A new stroke volume equation for thoracic electrical bioimpedance: theory and rationale. *Crit Care Med* 1986; **14**: 904–9.

15 Sherwood A, Carter LS Jr, Murphy CA. Cardiac output by impedance cardiography: two alternative methodologies compared with thermodilution. *Aviat Space Environ Med* 1991; **62**: 116–22.

16 Thomas SH. Impedance cardiography using the Sramek-Bernstein method: accuracy and variability at rest and during exercise. *Brit J Clin Pharmacol* 1992; **34**: 467–76.

17 Masaki DI, Greenspoon JS, Ouzounian JG. Noninvasive determination of cardiac output by thoracic electrical bioimpedance. *Crit Care Med* 1990; **18**: 121–2.

18 O'Connell AJ, Tibballs J, Coulthard M. Improving agreement between thoracic bioimpedance and dye dilution cardiac output estimation in children. *Anaesth Intens Care* 1991; **19**: 434–40.

19 Geddes LA, Sadler C. The specific resistance of blood at body temperature. *Med Biol Eng* 1973; **11**: 336–9.

20 Mohapatra SN, Costeloe KT, Hill DW. Blood resistivity and its implications for the calculation of cardiac output by the thoracic electrical impedance technique. *Intens Care Med* 1977; **3**: 63–7.

21 Quail AW, Traugott FM, Porges WL, White SW. Thoracic resistivity for stroke volume calculation in impedance cardiography. *J Appl Physiol* 1981; **50**: 191–5.

22 Thomas A, Vohra A, Pollard B. The effect of haematocrit on transthoracic electrical impedance and on the calculation of cardiac output by an impedance cardiograph. *Intens Care Med* 1991; **17**: 178–80.

23 Saladin V, Zussa C, Riscia G, Michielon P, Paccagnella A, Cipolotti G, *et al.* Comparison of cardiac output estimation by thoracic electrical bioimpedance, thermodilution, and Fick methods. *Crit Care Med* 1988; **16**: 1157–8.

24 Northridge DB, Findlay IN, Wilson J, Henderson E, Dargie HJ. Non-invasive determination of cardiac output by Doppler echocardiography and electrical impedance. *Brit Heart J* 1990; **63**: 93–7.

25 Aust PE, Belz GG, Koch W. Comparison of impedance cardiography and echocardiography for measurement of stroke volume. *Eur J Pharmacol* 1982; **23**: 475–77.

26 Loeppky JA, Hoekenga DA, Greene ER, Luft UC. Comparison of noninvasive pulsed Doppler and Fick measurements of stroke volume in cardiac patients. *Am Heart J* 1984; **107**: 339–46.

27 Hatcher DD, Srb OD. Comparison of two non-invasive techniques for estimating cardiac output during exercise. *J Appl Physiol* 1986; **61**: 155–9.

28 Smith SA, Russell AE, West MJ, Chalmers J. Automated non-invasive measurement of cardiac output: comparison of electrical bioimpedance and carbon dioxide rebreathing techniques. *Brit Heart J* 1988; **59**: 292–8.

29 Fuller HD. The validity of cardiac output measurement by thoracic impedance: a meta-analysis. *Clin Invest Med* 1992; **15**: 103–12.

30 Wong DH, Onishi R, Tremper KK, Reeves C, Zaccari J, Wong AB, *et al.* Thoracic bioimpedance and Doppler cardiac output measurement: learning curve and interobserver reproducibility. *Crit Care Med* 1989; **17**: 1194–8.

31 White SW, Quail AW, de Leeuw PW, Traugott FM, Brown WJ, Porges WL, *et al.* Impedance cardiography for cardiac output measurement: an evaluation of accuracy and limitations. *Eur Heart J* 1990; **11** (Suppl. I): 79–92.

32 Pickett BR, Buell JC. Validity of cardiac output measurement by computer-averaged impedance cardiography, and comparison with simultaneous thermodilution determinations. *Amer J Cardiol* 1992; **69**: 1354–8.

33 Ovsyshcher I, Gross JN, Blumberg S, Andrews C, Ritacco R, Furman S. Variability of cardiac output as determined by impedence cardiography in pacemaker patients. *Amer J Cardiol* 1993; **72**: 183–7.

34 Gotshall RW, Sexson WR. Comparison of band and spot electrodes for the measurement of stroke volume by the bioelectric impedance technique. *Crit Care Med* 1994; **22**: 420–5.

35 Mehlsen J, Bonde J, Stadeager C, Rehling M, Tango M, Trap-Jensen J. Reliability of impedance cardiography in measuring central haemodynamics. *Clin Physiol* 1991; **11**: 579–88.

36 Jensen L, Yakimets J, Teo KK. A review of impedance cardiography. *Heart Lung* 1995; **24**: 183–93.

37 Jewkes C, Sear JW, Verhoeff F, Sanders DJ, Foëx P. Non-invasive measurement of cardiac output by thoracic electrical bioimpedance: a study of reproducibility and comparison with thermodilution. *Brit J Anaesth* 1991; **67**: 788–94.

38 Yakimets J, Jensen L. Evaluation of impedance cardiography: comparison of NCCOM3-R7 with Fick and thermodilution methods. *Heart Lung* 1995; **24**: 194–206.

39 Duma S, Polzer K, Schlick W, Schuhfried F, Spiss C. Control of spontaneous respiration with continuous positive airway pressure using transthoracic electrical impedance. Studies in subjects with healthy lungs. *Anaesthesist* 1988; **37**: 218–23.

40 Woo MA, Hamilton M, Stevenson LW, Vredevoe DL. Comparison of thermodilution and transthoracic electrical bioimpedance cardiac outputs. *Heart Lung* 1991; **20**: 357–62.

41 Sageman WS, Amundson DE. Thoracic electrical bioimpedance measurement of cardiac output in postaortocoronary bypass patients. *Crit Care Med* 1993; **21**: 1139–42.

42 Miles DS, Cox MH, Verde TJ, Gotshall RW. Application of impedance cardiography during exercise. *Biol Psychol* 1993 **36**: 119–29.

43 Patterson R, Wang L, McVeigh G, Burns R, Cohn J. Impedance cardiography: the failure of sternal electrodes to predict changes in stroke volume. *Biol Psychol* 1993; **36**: 33–41.

44 Moon JK, Coggan AR, Hopper MK, Baker LE, Coyle EF. Stroke volume measurement during supine and upright cycle exercise by impedance cardiography. *Ann Biomed Eng* 1994; **22**: 514–23.

45 Antonicelli R, Savonitto S, Gambini C, Tomassini PF, Sardina M, Paciaroni E. Impedance cardiography for repeated determination of stroke volume in elderly hypertensives: correlation with pulsed Doppler echocardiography. *Angiology* 1991; **42**: 648–53.

46 Bowling LS, Sageman WS, O'Connor SM, Cole R, Amundson DE. Lack of agreement between measurement of ejection fraction by impedance cardiography versus radionuclide ventriculography. *Crit Care Med* 1993; **21**: 1523–7.

47 Boldt J, Kling D, Thiel A, Hempelmann G. Non-invasive versus invasive cardiovascular monitoring. Determination of stroke volume and pulmonary hydration using a new bioimpedance monitor. *Anaesthesist* 1988; **37**: 218–23.

48 Spinale FG, Reines HD, Cook MC, Crawford FA. Noninvasive estimation of extravascular lung water using bioimpedance. *J Surg Res* 1989; **47**: 535–40.

49 Woo EJ, Hua P, Webster JG, Tompkins WJ. Measuring lung resistivity using electrical impedance tomography. *IEEE Trans Biomed Eng* 1992; **39**: 756–60.

50 Donovan KD, Dobb GJ, Woods WPD, Hockings BE. Comparison of transthoracic electrical impedance and thermodilution methods for measuring cardiac output. *Crit Care Med* 1986; **14**: 1038–44.

51 Thomas SH, Molyneux P, Kelly J, Smith SE. The cardiovascular effects of oral nifedipine and nicardipine: a double-blind comparison in healthy volunteers using transthoracic bioimpedance cardiography. *Eur J Clin Pharmacol* 1990; **39**: 233–40.

52 World MJ. Estimation of cardiac output by bioimpedance cardiography. *J Roy Army Med Corps* 1990; **136**: 92–9.

53 Perrino AC Jr, Lippman A, Ariyan C, O'Connor TZ, Luther M. Intraoperative cardiac output monitoring: comparison of impedance cardiography and thermodilution. *J Cardiothorac Anesth* 1994; **8**: 24–9.

54 Shoemaker WC, Appel PL, Kram HB, Nathan RC, Thompson JL. Comparison of measurements of cardiac output by bioimpedance and thermodilution in severely ill surgical patients. *Crit Care Med* 1986; **14**: 933–5.

55 Preiser JC, Daper A, Parquier JN, Contempre B, Vincent JL. Transthoracic electrical bioimpedance versus thermodilution technique for cardiac output measurement during mechanical ventilation. *Intens Care Med* 1989; **15**: 221–3.

56 Spahn DR, Schmid ER, Torni CM, Jenni R, Segesser LV, Turina M, et al. Noninvasive versus invasive assessment of cardiac output after cardiac surgery: clinical validation. *J Cardiothor Anaesth* 1990; **4**: 46–59.

57 Belik J, Pelech A. Thoracic electric bioimpedance measurement of cardiac output in the newborn infant. *J Pediatr* 1988; **113**: 890–5.

58 Introna RP, Pruett JK, Crumrine RC, Cuadrado AR. Use of transthoracic bioimpedance to determine cardiac output in pediatric patients. *Crit Care Med* 1988; **16**: 1101–5.

59 Tibballs J. A comparative study of cardiac output in neonates supported by mechanical ventilation: measurement with thoracic electrical bioimpedance and pulsed Doppler ultrasound. *J Pediatr* 1989; **114**: 632–5.

60 Mickell JJ, Lucking SE, Chaten FC, Young ES. Trending of impedance-monitored cardiac variables: method and statistical power analysis of 100 control studies in a pediatric intensive care unit. *Crit Care Med* 1990; **18**: 645–50.

61 Sackner MA, Hoffman RA, Stroh D, Krieger BP. Thoracocardiography. Part 1: Noninvasive measurement of changes in stroke volume: comparisons to thermodilution. *Chest* 1991; **99**: 613–22. (See also Sackner MA, Hoffman RA, Krieger BP, Shaukat M, Stroh D, Sackner JD. Thoracocardiography. Part 2: Noninvasive measurement of changes in stroke volume: comparisons to impedance cardiography. *Chest* 1991; **99**: 896–903.)

62 Young JD, McQuillan P. Comparison of thoracic electrical bioimpedance and thermodilution for the measurement of cardiac index in patients with severe sepsis. *Brit J Anaesth* 1993; **70**: 58–62.

63 Thomas AN, Ryan J, Doran BRH, Pollard BJ. Bioimpedance versus thermodilution cardiac output measurement: the Bomed NCCOM3 after coronary bypass surgery. *Intens Care Med* 1991; **17**: 383–6.

64 Castor G, Molter G, Helms J, Niedermark I, Altmayer P. Determination of cardiac output during positive end-expiratory pressure – noninvasive electrical bioimpedance compared with standard thermodilution. *Crit Care Med* 1990; **18**: 544–6.

65 Shoemaker WC, Wo CC, Bishop MH, Appel PL, Van de Water JM, Harrington GR, *et al.* Multicenter trial of a new thoracic electrical bioimpedance device for cardiac output estimation. *Crit Care Med* 1994; **22**: 1907–12.

66 Balestra B, Malacrida R, Leonardi L, Suter P, Marone C. Esophageal electrodes allow precise assessment of cardiac output by bioimpedance. *Crit Care Med* 1992; **20**: 62–7.

67 Myhrman P, Granerus G, Karlsson K, Lundgren Y. Cardiac output in normal pregnancy measured by impedance cardiography. *Scand J Clin Lab Invest* 1982; **42**: 513–20.

68 Wong DH, Tremper KK, Stemmer EA, O'Connor D, Wilbur S, Zaccari J, *et al.* Noninvasive cardiac output: simultaneous comparison of two different methods with thermodilution. *Anesthesiology* 1990; **72**: 784–92.

69 Fein A, Grossman RF, Jones JG, Goodman PC, Murray JF. Evaluation of transthoracic electrical impedance in the diagnosis of pulmonary edema. *Circulation* 1979; **60**: 1156–60.

70 Saunders CF. The use of transthoracic electrical bioimpedance in assessing thoracic fluid status in emergency department patients. *Amer J Emerg Med* 1988; **6**: 337–40.

71 IEC 601–1 (EN 60601–1; BS 5724, Pt. 1). *General requirements for the safety of medical electrical equipment.* Geneva: International Electrotechnical Commission, 1988.

72 IEC 930. *Guidance for administrative, medical, and nursing staff concerned with the safe use of medical electrical equipment.* Geneva: International Electrotechnical Commission, 1988.

73 Hull CJ. The electrical hazards of patient monitoring. In: Hutton P, Prys-Roberts C, eds. *Monitoring in anaesthesia and intensive care.* London: W.B. Saunders Co, 1994: 56–77.

15 Alarms

General discussion of alarms philosophy

It is often assumed that virtually every variable sensed, displayed or recorded by a monitor, will be accompanied by alarms which will sound or visually alert in the event of a substantial variation from the norm. This is not necessarily the case, as the need for an attendant to be alerted should bear some relationship to the gravity of the change or event,[1] especially in so far as it might threaten the safety or well-being of the subject. It is easy to imagine that the cessation of the ECG signal and its displayed trace, for example, denotes cardiac arrest although, as discussed in Chapter 3, that might, in fact, not be the case. Nonetheless, the clinical circumstances which provoked the monitoring in the first place would tend to support the probability that such a change should be accompanied by an alarm to alert the attendant.

The need for an alarm in the case of other variables, in our case cardiovascular variables, may not be so obvious. If the blood pressure should change by a given amount or fall to a certain level, should the clinician or nurse be alerted immediately, or would it be safe for time to be allowed to elapse and the variable again measured? By this time, it might be clear whether a trend had been established or the real, potential, or perhaps spurious, problem was no longer present. Similarly, transient changes occur, sometimes substantially outside the limits that the user might accept as normal or reasonable in the clinical circumstances which are of no lasting importance. An example might be the sudden increase in blood pressure cuff pressure which occurs when it is momentarily disturbed or leaned upon during anaesthesia and surgery. Such transient changes are responsible for a proportion of spurious or "false" alarms. False alarms are important,[2] on account of the psychological effect that they have on those who must work with the equipment in which they are activated. False alarms cause irritation when they interrupt thought patterns or specific activities, both of which may be important at a given time, for example, when dealing with emergencies, in the care of the critically ill, and during the management of critical periods in anaesthesia. Estimates have been made of the prevalence of false alarms in particular settings: in the case of heart rate and blood pressure monitors, around 70% are believed to be false, about 15% to be of real significance and 1% to indicate life-threatening circumstances.[3-5]

It is not only false alarms which annoy and undermine the true attainable benefits of alarms. The very prevalence of alarm signals distributed among a variety of diagnostic and therapeutic equipment and monitors makes the annunciation of true alarms also a potent source of noise pollution for patients and those who have care of them.[6-27] It is estimated that more than 30 alarms are capable of sounding, some of them simultaneously, in a medium-sized special care baby unit, and there may be other devices in the cupboard which could be brought out at any moment. In the operating suite, an anaesthesia machine or workstation could produce between 20 and 50 different alarms,[28] some of which would refer to the same clinical activating condition. The position is worse in critical care areas,[29] where multiple therapeutic devices, each with an independent alarm, for example syringe drivers, infusion pumps, and controllers, are increasingly put to work in arrays of such devices without any intercommunication. Multiple alarms are not always needed in these circumstances and it may be the function, rather than the instrument, which requires the primary alarm.

A consequence of too frequent interruption by alarms, often accompanied by a high incidence of false alarms,[4] impels attendants to switch them off, where that is possible, to silence them,[3,7,9,11,30,31] or to take measures to alter or circumvent the alarm settings initially considered most appropriate. Moreover, the auditory characteristics of many medical alarm signals make them unduly intrusive[32] and add to the stimulus to dispense with them at the first opportunity. The foregoing may be summarised as too many alarms[3,9,14] with offensive sound characteristics, producing a cacaphony[33] at the expense of attendant and patient. The situation has been truly "alarming".[34,35] It would be simple to declare that only the most demanding situations should be allowed to provoke an alarm and that all other alarms should be suppressed.[36] Unfortunately, this counsel ignores the fact that many medical alarms and alarm systems are still too primitive to permit such an approach, so that some important alarms might never be annunciated.

It may be helpful to describe the problems surrounding the design and implementation of alarms in a number of specific respects, and to consider what improvements could be made. In some instances serious attempts at improvement have been made, but progress in the field has been slow.

What is the purpose of the alarm?

In the medical equipment setting, an alarm is intended to gain the attention of the user.[17,37-39] It is important to appreciate that the user may be assumed to have a certain amount of insight into the conditions in which the alarm may be expected to be activated; that the putative respondent may therefore be expected to have some knowledge of the equipment and its application; and that this respondent will have had appropriate training and experience in the field of use.[40] It is thus already quite different from the fire alarm or factory whistle.

A secondary purpose of an alarm in the monitoring setting is to enhance the vigilance of the attendant,[38] although care must be taken that the presence or availability of alarms does not promote false confidence that the alarm system will take care of the patient with a consequent decrease in vigilance.

What is expected of the respondent to the alarm?

Given the above, it would seem unnecessary to attract the respondent's attention in an unduly dramatic fashion. Further, the means need not be intrusive or offensive, provided it is easily recognisable by a person of such training and experience. The alarm need not then persist in a form which intrudes into thought processes or decision-making once its presence and validity have been recognised.[36] Hence, the respondent should be in a position to respond appropriately to alarms which convey the necessary basic information in a form germane to the application and convenient to the respondent.

Medical alarms and the responses expected

Purpose

- Gain the attention of the attendant (respondent)
- Enhance vigilance in the attendant

Response expected

- Attendant should be in a position to appreciate the significance of the implied warning
- The alarm should alert only those for whom it is intended (i.e. *not* alarm those it does not concern)
- Response should be appropriate to its priority and urgency

What form might the alarm take?

Alarms may be conveniently divided into those which are audible and those which are visible. Common usage and convention have determined that these be known as "auditory" and "visual" alarms. Hitherto, some information heralded by alarms has been simply informative and need not be visited upon the respondent in the form of an alarm as such. Simple, recognisable sounds, dedicated to preceding information only, may be termed information sounds.

Categories of medical alarm sounds

Annunciation

- Visual
- Auditory

Urgency

- High priority (warning)
- Medium priority (cautionary)
- Low priority (attention)
- Information

It has been proposed that the nature of the alarm should be determined by the urgency of the situation to which the host monitor is applied. The widespread conception (or misconception) of the term "alarm" when applied in the clinical setting has therefore prompted the signals produced by monitors and other medical equipment being referred to as warning, cautionary, attention, and information sounds, whose priority – high, medium or low – reflects the degree of urgency. The levels of priority are: *high priority*, implying that the condition provoking the alarm requires an immediate response; *medium priority*, where the condition is potentially serious or dangerous and demands a prompt response; and *low priority*, which indicates that awareness is necessary on the part of the respondent.[36] The corresponding auditory signals are termed *warning* signal, *cautionary* signal, and *attention* signal, respectively. Auditory alarms are believed to attract attention more readily than visual signals,[41] albeit at the price of greater intrusiveness. It has been stated that manufacturers may deliberately make their alarms excessively intrusive, so as to absolve themselves of blame in the event of a poor outcome and thus transfer responsibility from the device to the user.[42] As the practice of medicine becomes more dependent on device technology, the attention of clinicians, nurses, and others concerned with the well-being of the patient, is diverted to specific tasks which may consume much their concentration,[43] so that they are unable to keep a wholly constant watch on the whole patient and the monitors. Alarms then serve the very useful function of attracting attention to the abnormal, where the normal may reasonably safely be ignored for the stated compelling reasons.

Information signals would not necessarily evoke an overt response. It is equally important to note that low, medium, and even high priority alarms might not appear to provoke a physical response from the attendant, as the first response may justifiably be a rapid assessment of the alarm and its circumstances, whereupon one of the considered clinical options may be simply to do nothing.

Possible responses to alarm annunciation

Recognise the warning
Assess its significance and urgency (priority)
On the basis of that assessment and *as appropriate*:

- act now
  or
- defer action in the light of present commitment
  or
- do nothing (no overt action for the time being)*

* Note. A clear distinction must be drawn between: ignoring a warning, and noting the warning but deciding that instant action is unnecessary or inappropriate.

Are alarms really necessary?

Whatever the background philosophy, real world events now dictate that those who carry out procedures that might in any way harm the patient inadvertently should be seen to be exercising due care and attention. Common sense suggests that the mere presence of alarms is not the solution if they go unheeded or the manner of their implementation encourages their sporadic use or abandonment. However, the constant threat of litigation, especially in the USA,[44] has led to medical insurance premiums being strongly influenced by the adoption of recommendations, protocols, and checklists for monitoring and monitoring equipment, and associated alarms.[45-49] In support of the concept, it has been shown that monitoring standards sometimes fall short in practice;[50-52] that human error is indeed very much with us;[53-55] that fatigue due to long hours[56] and disrupted sleep patterns[57] does impair performance,[58,59] and that monitors and alarms could help prevent the untoward consequences.[41,49,53,60-64] The stress of some occupations has also been shown to contribute to poor performance[65] and it has been demonstrated that truly constant vigilance is an ideal rarely attained.[66] The logging of alarms as they occur, together with logging of significant events recorded by monitoring systems has been recommended in the light of suspected interference with equipment.[40] Alarm and data logging can make a substantial contribution to the audit of performance by those using therapeutic and monitoring equipment and by those responsible

203

both for standards of care and practice in institutions and elsewhere, and in the arbitration and settlement of claims. It is at the same time urged that standards of monitoring, being in fashion, may be proliferating excessively and should be accepted with some care,[67] and that too much reliance on monitors may lead to loss of competence in clinical methods.[50,52,68]

Standards for alarm signals

The requirements for alarm signals for medical equipment have been defined in European Standard (CEN) EN 475.[69] Similar international (ISO) standards, so far restricted to anaesthetic and respiratory equipment, are ISO 9703–1[70] and ISO 9703–2[71] for visual and auditory signals, respectively. There is a separate, but similar, American Standard, ASTM-F1463–93.[72]

Visual warning signals

The visual alarm (or, in standards terms, visual warning signal) standards specify the colours to be used and their duty cycles (that is, the period for which they are on and off or flashing). They demand, for example, that the colour green be used only to show that the equipment or function is in a state of readiness for use, whilst flashing red and yellow are used for the warning and cautionary signals, and continuous yellow for the attention signal.

Visual warning signals have the virtue of being non-intrusive when displayed. It is therefore useful for them to persist during the period of active response, during subsequent assessment and management, and as reminders in the event of distraction. However, visual warning signals alone may go unnoticed, or may be difficult to see from certain vantage points or when the respondent is engrossed in a particular task.[73] If sounds are difficult to locate, a light used as a general beacon may help identify the instrument/monitor cluster responsible for alarm annunciation. Illuminated displays may also carry limited or more liberal information as to their nature and purpose. Information displays, as exemplified by liquid crystal displays (LCD), other illuminated panels, and cathode-ray oscilloscope (CRT) screens, are generally exempt from the colour restrictions.

Auditory warning signals

The nature of the recommended sounds warrants discussion. The auditory warning signal should have characteristics that are of value to its

Visual alarm signals

Colours*

- Green – signifies the equipment is switched on and ready for use
- Yellow (continuous) – requires the attention of the operator/respondent
- Yellow (flashing) – indicates that caution is necessary
- Red (flashing) – indicates a warning
- Any other colour – information only

Note: dot-matrix and similar displays, as for example on CRTs, are exempt from the colour requirements.

Duty cycle and flashing frequency

- Duty cycle is the proportion of time on in each cycle (20–60% in each case)
- Flashing occurs at the frequency specified in the Standard

Relationship with auditory alarms

- Auditory *warning* (high priority) signals must be accompanied by the corresponding visual signal, which must be flashing red if a light is used
- Auditory *cautionary* (medium priority) signals need not be accompanied by the corresponding visual signal – if they are, it must be flashing yellow
- There is no obligatory auditory component in the *attention* (low priority signal) – it is visual indication which, if a light is used, is continuous yellow and which may or may not be accompanied by the low priority audible signal
- Information signals consist of an auditory signal or a visual indication, or both, and any auditory component must not have the characteristics of warning or cautionary signals, and unless an alphanumeric or computer graphic display is used the visual indication must not be red

particular users. It should not startle; it should not be unduly loud, strident all-pervasive, or continuous; it should be audible in a range of conditions; and it should convey the degree of urgency. It should also be locatable and recognisable, and not easily confused with competing but unrelated sounds, such as machinery, personal pagers, door chimes, and the like.

Startle reactions are not confined to the attendants but, especially in critical care areas, is germane to the patients within earshot. Any sound which is generally identifiable as a crude alarm sound may be recognised as such by any of the patients in the vicinity, some of whom cannot know that it does not refer to them. Similarly, such sounds are also likely to distress relatives and other visitors who may be concerned about anyone to whom they believe the alarm might refer. Very loud sounds may inhibit constructive thought, especially if loud and strident.[74,75]

Auditory alarm signals

Pulses are the building blocks of the auditory alarm signal
- Gentle onset (non-startling) and gentle release
- Broad frequency band (to avoid confusion with other sounds and to assist in localisation)

Bursts comprise groups of pulses so as to convey the sense of priority of the audible signal

Sounds
- Warning (high priority) signal: has the general characteristics shown in Figure 15.1 (a), consists of a double burst as in Figure 15.1 (c) of five pulses, and is accompanied by a visual indication (flashing red if a light is used)
- Cautionary (medium priority) signal: has the general characteristics shown in Figure 15.1 (a), consists of a single burst as in Figure 15.1 (b) of three pulses, and is accompanied by a visual indication (flashing yellow if a light is used)
- Attention (low priority) signal: when used, has the general characteristics shown in Figure 15.1 (a), consists of a single burst as in Figure 15.1 (c) of one or more pulses
- Information signal: must not have the characteristics of the warning or cautionary signals

Notes:

1 The high priority (warning) and medium priority (cautionary) audible signals are distinguished by the double or single burst and the number of pulses in the burst.
2 The pitch of the pulses in high and medium priority bursts may change in steps between the first and last pulses, but the change must be in one direction only – it may also change in low priority bursts of more than one pulse, but with no restriction on direction
3 These characteristics are quite different from those of conventional public alarms, such as fire alarms and sirens, as they are aimed at a distinct set of trained respondents and need not alarm or alert others.

Indeed, the first reaction may not be to analyse the conditions which may have provoked the alarm, but to seek to silence or attenuate it, thereby losing both thinking time and concentration. As already mentioned, once the audible alarm is appreciated, there is no reason to persist with it unless it is not acknowledged. Hence, a brief annunciation of a non-startling, characteristic and not unduly loud sound repeated at intervals will suffice, thereby satisfying the practical requirement that an audible alarm, once annunciated and recognised, should be silenced.[36]

Suitable sounds can be specified as a "pulse" of sound characterised by a graphical envelope whose parameters are pulse amplitude and duration

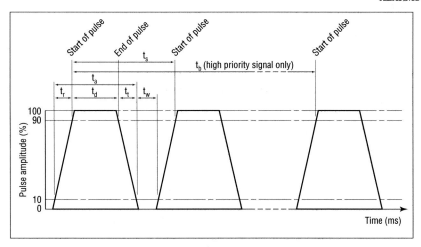

Figure 15.1(a) Temporal characteristics of auditory medical alarm signals. t_b = burst spacing; t_d = effective pulse duration; t_f = pulse fall time; t_o = overall pulse duration; t_r = pulse rise time; t_s = pulse spacing; t_w = pulse spacing width. Redrawn from Temporal characteristics of auditory signals (CEN EN, p. 9, Fig. 1).

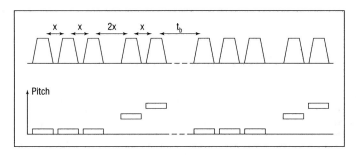

Figure 15.1(b) A high priority (warning) sound burst of pulses. (top) There are five pulses in the burst. X = a fixed value ($\pm 5\%$) between 150 ms and 250 ms; t_b = (2.0 + 0.2) s. The effective pulse duration (t_d) is 150 to 200 ms, and both rise and fall times are 10%–20% of t_d. The amplitude of pulses may be between 45 and 85 dB(A), but the difference in amplitude between any two pulses must not exceed 10 dB(A). The double burst may be repeated at intervals of (10 ± 2.5) s (unless otherwise specified in the Particular Standard for a particular medical device). (bottom) The pitch of successive pulses in a burst may be the same as or higher or lower than that of its predecessor. However, if any pulse has a pitch higher than any preceding pulse in the burst, then any succeeding pulse must have a pitch that is the same as or higher than the pulse in question. Similarly, any pulse of a lower pitch than a predecessor can only be followed by a pulse of the same or a lower pitch than itself. That is, any change in pitch within a burst can only proceed in the same direction, so that change within the pulse is perceived as rising or falling but not both. Redrawn from Double burst (based on extraction from CEN EN 475, p. 9, Fig. 1).

(Figure 15.1a). Each pulse has the non-startling, locatable, recognisable and attention-attracting properties referred to, whilst the pulses are gathered together in a "burst", the number and temporal spacing of which indicate the urgency of the warning signal (Figure 14.1b and c).

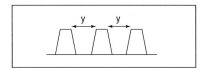

Figure 15.1(c) A medium priority (cautionary) sound burst of pulses. There are three pulses in the burst. Y=a fixed value (±5%) between 250 ms and 500 ms. The effective pulse duration (t_d) is 150 to 200 ms, and both rise and fall times are 10%–20% of t_d. The amplitude of pulses may be between 45 and 85 dB (A), but the difference in amplitude between any two pulses must not exceed 10 dB (A). The single burst may be repeated at intervals of (25±5) s (unless otherwise specified in the Particular Standard for a particular medical device). The pitch of successive pulses in a burst may be the same as or higher than or lower than that of its predecessor. The requirements concerning any change in pitch within a burst are as for the high priority sound (see Fig. 15.1 b). Redrawn from Structure of burst (based on extraction from CEN EN 475, p. 9, Fig.1).

The implementation of alarms is the province of standards specifying the characteristics of particular items of medical equipment. Ideally, a period of silence would occur automatically after annunciation but, should the alarm be ignored or forgotten under the pressure of a demanding workload, it would recur at intervals until properly dealt with, rather than sounding continuously as is almost always the case at present. Here is an excellent opportunity for reducing both noise pollution and stress occasioned by the needless prevalence of alarm sounds. In addition, if the signal were not acknowledged, the apparent urgency of the signal might be increased by temporal compression of the separated bursts or by a change in priority, as in a so-called "scalable" alarm.

The almost universal notion of what an alarm should sound like, mentioned at the start of this chapter, proved a considerable obstacle to the acceptance of the improved sounds, since they were "not proper alarms" and did not really sound like the "tunes" which are frequently suggested as a solution to the problems of identification. Indeed, the sounds seem quite innocuous to those whom they do not concern; do not distract, amuse or appear faintly ridiculous (as "tunes" in such circumstances inevitably do); and are identifiable by those who have been informed of their existence and instructed in their use.

The original work on these sounds, conducted in the UK, was based on the work of Patterson[76,77] and his colleagues at the MRC Applied Psychology Unit, Cambridge. They had successfully devised sounds for civil aircraft,[78] where there were similar problems and the previous alarms had many of the shortcomings identified in the medical field. The nature of the required alarm sounds and the circumstances in which they are annunciated in the cockpit and on the flight-deck, however, are significantly different from the medical requirements, although based on the same basic principles.[79,80] For example, the duplication and triplication of equipment and monitors (redundancy) in modern aircraft, together with attempts to process data such that only a few highly informative, coherent and coordinated displays are necessary,[81] thus reducing what has been called pilot overload,[82] is far removed from the position in medical applications. There, many different devices, usually standing alone, from different manufacturers and monitoring quite different variables in different disciplines, is the rule. A new set of alarm sounds appropriate to these conditions was therefore devised by a team which included clinicians and nurses with immediate experience of the disciplines and environments concerned.

It is reasonable to question the need for the newer sounds, since many clinicians and nurses would submit that they become expert in detecting the alarm sounds emitted by the equipment with which they happen to be familiar, and in differentiating between conflicting current alarms. Such studies as there are do not confirm this belief.[73,83-85] Moreover, they may experience difficulty when they encounter new equipment or move to new clinical environments.

Further field testing of the new sounds should confirm or refute the claims in respect of substantial improvement in recognition, but preliminary experiments conducted with groups of nurses and others, including some consisting of highly trained intensive care nurses, have shown that the sounds are easily memorised in the first instance and retained throughout continuous experience, and are relearned very readily after lapses in continuous exposure. It has been shown also that personnel who habitually work with medical devices and monitoring equipment can learn up to 10 distinct varieties of bursts of pulses. The UK proposals initially contained six such sounds for six sets of circumstances, viz. "ventilation", "oxygenation", "cardiovascular", "artificial perfusion", "drug administration" and "temperature", which it was believed would cover foreseeable circumstances in medical practice. One authority proposed that the introduction of sets of new sounds would make a bad situation worse,[86] although this view seemed to be based on the assumption that some or all of the sounds might be activated simultaneously. In fact, the overall work programme for alarm standards envisages guidance on the implementation of alarms in given types of therapeutic and monitoring equipment, which would recommend prioritisation and other measures enabling a competent designer to avoid such obvious pitfalls. It appears that the climate of opinion may be changing as progress is made, but the final outcome remains to be seen. The sounds in the European standard apply to medical equipment generally so that, when implemented, they should be uniform throughout all sites and disciplines in hospital, community, and home applications.

The specifications published in the standard are somewhat less rigorous than those originally submitted and represent a compromise between what may seem ideal and what manufacturers feel able to accept at present. Initially, there was resistance also on the grounds of complexity of the circuitry and cost, but recent developments have reduced both very substantially. It is often argued that small devices, the simplicity and engineering elegance of which enable them to be sold inexpensively, cannot be equipped with anything more than the smallest and least costly alarm unit. It can equally be urged that alarms should be commensurate with the degree of risk faced by the patient and attendant and, given the current state-of-the-art and predicted improvements, alarms should be awarded their rightful design priority.

A common problem in intensive care and special care baby units is the difficulty of locating sounds that, because of low ceilings, sound-reflective walls, pillars, screens and mobile shelf units, may be very difficult to pin-point. The sounds may also share characteristics with sounds of lesser importance but which have been designed for more general use (for example, personal pagers), for low-level summonses to attention (door chimes), or in advance of public information announcements. Other machinery and devices used in the operating suite, critical care areas, and general wards and departments, and even in the community and at home, may share the frequencies of crude alarms and render them inaudible by virtue of auditory masking.[87] Many of the alarms built into even complex life-saving devices have been the least expensive, off-the-shelf buzzers or sounders available. The solution to both of these problems lies in the harmonic content of the sound, that is, providing a sound containing a number of different frequencies. In the case of sound reflection, the different frequencies are reflected unequally, thereby leading the respondent to the source. If the frequencies are chosen judiciously, the sound itself need not be loud to be eminently discernible and locatable. These features are covered in the standard alarm sounds specifications.

The question of urgency presents itself differently in different disciplines. Where a monitor subserves a single function or set of functions as in, for example, an infusion pump or controller, the information needed by the respondent concerns only the degree of urgency tied to the particular function or functions. However, if the monitor subserves several different functions, especially where they are unrelated, the position becomes more difficult. Many monitoring assemblies supplied for use in critical care or anaesthesia contain a mixture of respiratory and cardiovascular modules with discrete or common alarms,[88,89] depending upon the particular design concept. The problem for the respondent now is not simply to identify the degree of urgency associated with one type of variable, but to determine the relative urgency of alarms if they are multiple or concern two unrelated variables, both of which may have important implications for the patient. Critical care units and, increasingly, some wards and departments, exemplify a more serious problem, in which the respondent, usually a nurse, is required to decide which alarm to attend to when more than one is activated at more than one treatment site. Does the nurse continue with an important task and attend the adjacent alarm site when ready, or must the task be abandoned in order to see just how serious the other alarm is? This problem of relative urgency between variables and the systems which they represent is complex and a cause of stress for the staff concerned. On the surface, the professional nurse may appear unruffled when coolly making such decisions, but nevertheless is continually exposed to knowing that the choice is often arbitrary and could prove unsound despite the best of motives.

The intermittent and relatively non-intrusive auditory alarm sound may be supported by a visual indication and, when the urgency enjoys a high priority, will always be supported by a continuous visual signal for as long as the high-priority condition persists or the alarms are discontinued.

Silencing of alarms

Many authorities believe that both visual and auditory alarms should not be capable of being disabled other than in clearly defined circumstances. However, as has been noted, unless the sounds are conducive to being well received and calmly acted upon, respondents will be inclined to disable them. The periodically activated sounds discourage this practice and permit the design of alarms which are only susceptible to silencing under defined and warranted conditions, including confirmation that the alarm has been acknowledged. Reasonable indications include silencing of alarms on start-up, while instrument testing, set-up, and calibration are carried out, and muting during specific therapeutic manoeuvres, where the otherwise inevitable alarm would serve only as a distraction. A suitable period might be no more than 120 seconds. It is important that, where an auditory alarm is silenced legitimately, the fact that the alarms are inoperative is indicated.

Alarm settings

It follows that the alarm settings must be determined manually or automatically in accordance with the need for an alarm, its activation in given circumstances, and its priority. In the absence of agreed standards or protocols,[90] it appears that alarm settings are the province of those who have responsibility for the care of the patient at that point; that is, the nurse or clinician in the critical care or emergency unit, the anaesthetist in the operating suite, or the nurse or paramedical staff member in wards, departments, and the community.

The incidence of false alarms for a given monitor may be instantly reduced by setting alarm limits to span a large range of values,[91,92] perhaps

Alarm settings

May be achieved manually or automatically

Manual

- Alarm limit setting is often a critical operation and should be performed with care
- Settings should be dedicated to the patient and condition
- Avoid arbitrary settings or settings simply handed down by tradition – think about them!
- Bear in mind who it is that will be expected to respond and what response is expected – it may not be you
- Avoid too "tight" (close) settings that will yield an excess of false alarms
- Avoid too wide settings – they will not catch problems until it is too late
- If there are locks or deterrents on the setting controls, use them
- Record the settings and any changes made to them

Automatic

- Are the settings always the same at switch-on, that is, are they "default" settings? *or* Are they carried over from the settings left by the previous user? If they can be – then check first and reset if necessary
- Can you exert your own user preference on default settings at start-up?
- Do the settings respond to results obtained from these or other monitored variables? It is important to know whether or not this is the case in your monitoring system.

outside the range of immediate concern. If so, many of the warnings will still be false,[92] and true warnings may be given only when matters have progressed beyond a point which is permissible and where the patient's condition may in any case be clinically obvious. Conversely, setting alarms to cover a very restricted range obviates this situation at the expense of many spurious alarms, thereby inducing a tendency for further alarms to be disregarded.[31,33] Introducing a delay between the sensing of an aberrant variable in a condition meriting an alarm and activating that alarm also reduces the incidence of false alarms,[9,93] but warnings requiring an immediate response will be recognised just that little bit later.

What is required, then, is a setting commensurate with the expected range of monitored values, the expected response of the attendant and, hence, the limits which are for the moment considered suitable thresholds for the activation of the alarm concerned. Extreme settings should be avoided.[33,43] All too commonly, alarms are left set at the manufacturer's default values[94] and not subsequently adjusted. It has been stated that manufacturers sometimes set default on the side of excessive caution for fear of the consequences of product liability legislation,[95] on the basis that false alarms cost less than missed events.[75] A problem connected with default values concerns the fact that, although many monitoring instruments start up with the manufacturer's default settings, others retain the settings from the previous use with no immediate indication that unusual limits are still in operation. A more insidious form of this is seen in circumstances where automated blood pressure monitors used in conjunction with anaesthetic machines or anaesthetic workstations quite reasonably retain the set limits (and indeed, the last recorded blood pressure values for the previous patient) between patients and there is no prompt to reset. Most suppliers of such apparatus do, however, have modes for recall of settings or permanent display of these, if required. The incorporation of scalable alarms, limits of which can be set automatically according to the values being recorded over a period for a given patient, is a likely development which calls for intelligent processing of data. False alarms also occur as the result of imperfect placing of sensors and electrodes and insecure fixing at the intended site. Care with these aspects again reduces their incidence.[96]

The settings themselves should be apparent to the respondent. When set by rotary controls, they need to be clearly visible and need not be in absolute numeric values and, in some instances, might better be indicated as the passing of some point or the breaching of some nominated condition of the monitor or its alarm. Thumb-wheels have been popular and have the advantage that they can be combined with displayed numerical values of the settings. Both rotary and thumb-wheel controls should be fitted with some sort of restraint, such as positive locks, baulks or detents, to prevent accidental movement. The increasing use of software controls, in the form of keypads and similar digital setting devices, introduces the possibility of accidental contact or erroneous operation. It is recommended that alarm settings, just as important equipment control settings, should be effected only by a definitive sequence of key presses or contacts, in order to reduce these possibilities.

In a recent report on alarms on monitoring equipment[40] resulting from problems arising in a paediatric setting, but addressing a wide range of important issues in monitoring and the associated alarms, it is recommended *inter alia* that alarm settings should be recorded, for example, in the patient's record. Such a practice, apart from its implications for good record-keeping and medicolegal purposes, would necessarily draw attention to the need for definitive alarm setting[97] and the need to undertake this for each case.

Prioritisation and enhancement (escalation) of (scalable) alarms

The problems surrounding multiple activation and annunciation of auditory alarms beg solutions. Much effort has been devoted to this, but has been hampered by the lack of commonly delineated approaches and the lack of interdevice communications standards. Many monitoring devices are provided with the popular RS-232 25-pin communications output socket.[98] However, in practice, some devices use only subsets of the pin-out and there are many variations on the allocations of the individual pins, with sometimes potentially serious consequences for the monitors and the equipment to which they are connected. It is therefore not a sufficiently robust standard for this purpose. A common communications pathway (or bus) is required. The Institute of Electrical and Electronic Engineers (IEEE, or "I-triple E", as is it often known) has been working on a medical information bus (MIB)[99] for a number of years and the first level has recently been published. It is based to some extent on a proprietary design and there are alternative proposals, although none of these has yet reached fruition. Working Group 5 of CEN European Standards committee CEN/ TC 251 (Medical Informatics) is working on draft standards for communications between medical devices and on the format of the data which would be exchanged between them.

Already single monitors and local monitoring arrays and systems have had their alarm signals "prioritised". One school of thought suggests that only the most important signal should be annunciated.[36] Another suggests that the alarm system should track a variable in order to activate it when danger threatens;[33] and others have suggested that the most important should be annunciated, followed by the next important (perhaps with a limit on the number of variables allowed in succession) with, of course, the mandatory periods of silence between bursts, an arrangement which has been referred to as priority interlocking.[100] An alternative approach is that a single system alarm burst subserves the needs of any or all variables requiring annunciation, and visual indicators provide information on the variables concerned and their absolute or relative degrees of urgency. The anaesthetic workstation has proved to be an attractive test-bed,[101] since several cardiovascular and respiratory variables are continuously monitored in well-recognised combinations, and several such machines have been placed on the commercial market. Experience is promising in this area and the principles would seem to be applicable to critical care, wards and departments but, as noted, progress is somewhat thwarted by the absence of standard buses, networks, and data formats.

A separate aspect of prioritisation concerns the ability of the attendant to predetermine change in the priority of an alarm, should the condition provoking it change or should its allocated priority become greater or less in relation to a newly annunciated alarm.[91] Thus, an example would be an alarm associated with heart rate and allocated medium priority being advanced to high priority status at a given threshold level; this itself might then become of a lesser priority in the event of a persistent low blood

214

pressure alarm. The priority of this, in turn, would be reduced when effective therapy restored a satisfactory blood pressure.

Intelligent monitoring and alarm systems

Intelligent alarms,[91,102–106] sometimes referred to as "smart" alarms, sample data generated by the monitor in order to capture extreme values, trends, and events and to evaluate these in order to:

- generate informative reports (visual or printed);
- analyse trends on more than one variable in order to generate alarms based on several interdependent variables, rather than just one;[107]
- adjust internal programming of machines, the normal working of which depends on software algorithms;
- make adjustments to alarm settings automatically as data sampling, display, and recording proceed.[108,109]

It is claimed that intelligent systems reduce alarm response times.[105] Various approaches can be used, including dedicated algorithms (that may become very complex);[110] analysis of probabilities;[1] fuzzy logic, rule-based,[111,112] neural networks,[113] and expert systems.[114,115] Consideration of these methods, which are finding application in many and diverse ways in clinical practice, is beyond the scope of this book.

Alarms for non-invasive cardiovascular monitoring

The preceding commentary applies to monitoring equipment in general, and non-invasive cardiovascular monitoring equipment shares the principle characteristics.

The electrocardiogram is commonly supplied with heart rate alarms, whilst advanced ECG monitors, ECG recorders, and arrythmia monitors and detectors may have alarms concerned with the detection of arrhythmias, undesirable trends during trace analysis, and actual and potential cardiac events. False alarms are commonly associated with poor quality, poorly sited, or poorly fixed electrodes, all of which problems are easily remedied.

Blood pressure monitoring is less clear-cut. Most equipment is provided with high and low alarms on the systolic blood pressure, but the significance of mean blood pressure and pulse pressure (the difference between systolic and diastolic pressures) is largely ignored. Moreover, many clinicians, nurses and others continue to use arbitrary values for alarm settings. Alarms set too close give frequent spurious alarms in the operating suite and the critical care area, whilst wide settings defeat the purpose of the alarms. Algorithms in automatic blood pressure monitors are being improved constantly and are capable of detecting many artefacts. However, unless respondents can be encouraged to set alarm limits with considerably more care than formerly, it might be concluded that blood pressure alarms are of limited value or, perhaps preferably, that intelligent alarm systems should be used which adjust initial default settings to the circumstances encountered during use and to trends predicted by analysis of pertinent data held in the monitoring device.

1 Beinlich IA, Gaba DM. The ALARM monitoring system – intelligent decision making under uncertainty. *Anesthesiology* 1989; **71**: A 337.
2 Kunz JC. *The occurrence of alarms in the ICU.* San Francisco: Institutes of Medical Science Report, 1976.
3 Kestin I, Miller B, Lockhart C. Auditory alarms during anesthesia monitoring. *Anesthesiology* 1988; **69**: 106–9.
4 Koski EM, Makivirta A, Sukuvaara T, Kari A. Frequency and reliability of alarms in the monitoring of cardiac postoperative patients. *Int J Clin Monit Comput* 1990; 7: 129–33.
5 Lawless ST. Crying wolf: false alarms in a pediatric intensive care unit. *Crit Care Med* 1994; **22**: 981–5.
6 Shapiro R, Berland T. Noise in the operating room. *New Engl J Med* 1972; **287**: 1236–38.
7 McIntyre J. Ergonomics: anaesthetists' use of auditory alarms in the operating room. *Int J Clin Monit Comput* 1985; **2**: 47–55.
8 O'Carroll T. Survey of alarms in an intensive therapy unit. *Anaesthesia* 1986; **41**: 742–4.
9 Schaaf C, Block FE. Evaluation of alarm sounds in the operating room. *J Clin Monit* 1989; **5**: 300–1.
10 Weinger M, Englund C. Ergonomic and human factors affecting anesthetic vigilance and monitoring performance in the operating room environment. *Anesthesiology* 1990; **73**: 995–1021.
11 McIntyre JW. Alarms in the operating room. *Can J Anaesth* 1991; **38**: 951–3.
12 Momtahan H, Hetu R, Tansley B. Audibility and identification of auditory alarms in the operating room and intensive care unit. *Ergonomics* 1993; **36**: 1159–76.
13 Weinger MB, Smith NT. Vigilance, alarms, and integrated monitoring systems. In: Ehrenwerth J, Eisenkraft JB, eds. *Anesthesia equipment: principles and applications.* St. Louis: CV Mosby, 1993.
14 Schulte GT, Block FE Jr. Can people hear the pitch on a variable-pitch pulse oximeter? *Anesthesiology* 1989; **70**: A340.
15 Bentley S, Murphy F, Dudley H. Perceived noise in surgical wards and intensive care area: an objective analysis. *BMJ* 1972; **3**: 1503–6.
16 Falk SA, Woods NF. Hospital noise-levels and potential health hazards. *New Engl J Med* 1973; **289**: 774–81.
17 Wellens HJ, Vermeulen A, Durrer D. Ventricular fibrillation occurring on arousal from sleep by auditory stimuli. *Circulation* 1972; **46**: 661–5.
18 Hilton BA. Quantity and quality of patients' sleep and sleep-disturbing factors in a respiratory intensive care unit. *J Adv Nurs* 1976; **1**: 453–68.
19 Smith R, Johnson L, Rothfield D. Sleep and cardiac arrhythmias. *Arch Int Med* 1972; **130**: 751–3.
20 Noble MA. Communication in ICU; therapeutic or distressing? *Nurs Outlook* 1979; **27**: 195–8.
21 Gloag D. Noise: hearing loss and psychological effects. *BMJ* 1980; **281**: 1325–7.
22 Hodge B, Thompson JF. Noise pollution in the operating theatre. *Lancet* 1990; **335**: 891–4.
23 Minckley BB. A study of noise and its relationship to patient discomfort in the recovery room. *Nurs Res* 1968; **17**: 247–50.
24 Hansell HN. The behavioural effects of noise on man: the patient with "intensive care psychosis". *Heart Lung* 1984; **13**: 59–65.
25 Hilton A. The hospital racket: how noisy is your unit? *Am J Nurs* 1987; **87**: 59–61.

26 Richards KC, Bairnsfather L. A description of night sleep patterns in the critical care unit. *Heart Lung* 1988; **17**: 35–42.

27 Topf M, David JE. Critical care unit noise and rapid eye movement (REM) sleep. *Heart Lung* 1993; **22**: 252–8.

28 Kam PCA, Kam AC, Thompson JF. Noise pollution in the anaesthetic and intensive care environment. *Anaesthesia* 1994; **49**: 982–6.

29 Cropp AJ, Woods LA, Raney D, Bredle DL. Name that tone. The proliferation of alarms in the intensive care unit. *Chest* 1994; **105**: 1217–20.

30 Kerr JH. Alarms and excursions. *Anaesthesia* 1986; **41**: 807–8.

31 Kerr JH. Warning devices. *Brit J Anaesth* 1985; **57**: 696–708.

32 Schmidt SI, Baysinger CL. Alarms: help or hindrance? *Anesthesiology* 1986; **64**: 654–5.

33 Bedford RF. Technology: Is it helping us or creating problems? *Proc NY State Soc Anesthesiologists Ann Postgrad Ass*, December 15, 1986, New York City: 211–12.

34 Kerr JH, Hayes B. An "alarming situation" in the intensive therapy unit. *Intens Care Med* 1983; **9**: 103–4.

35 Samuels SI. An alarming problem. *Anesthesiology* 1986; **64**: 128–9.

36 Schreiber P, Schreiber J. Structured alarm systems for the operating room. *J Clin Monit* 1989; **5**: 201–4.

37 Allnutt M. Human factors in accidents. *Br J Anaesth* 1987; **59**: 856–64.

38 Beneken JE, van der Aa JJ. Alarms and their limits in monitoring. *J Clin Monit* 1989; **5**: 210–15.

39 Quinn ML. Semipractical alarms: a parable. *J Clin Monit* 1989; **5**: 196–200.

40 *The report of the expert working group on alarms on clinical monitors*. London, Medical Devices Agency, 1995: pp. 11–23.

41 Morgan M. Editorial: a confidential inquiry into perioperative deaths. *Anaesthesia* 1988; **43**: 91–2.

42 Hayman W, Drinker P. Design of medical device alarm systems. *Med Instrum* 1983; **17**: 103–6.

43 Sykes MK. Panel on practical alarms: Fifth International Symposium on Computing in Anesthesia and Intensive Care. Introduction. *J Clin Monit* 1989; **5**: 192–3.

44 Zeitlin GL, Cass WA, Gessner JS. Insurance incentives and the use of monitoring devices. *Anesthesiology* 1988; **69**: 441.

45 *Recommendations for standards of monitoring during anaesthesia and recovery*. London: Association of Anaesthetists of Great Britain and Ireland, 1988 (revised edition 1994).

46 Eichhorn JH, Cooper JB, Cullen DJ, Maier WR, Philip JH, Seeman RG. Standards for patient monitoring during anesthesia at Harvard Medical School. *JAMA* 1986; **256**: 1017–20.

47 Quality assurance in anaesthesiology. Guidelines of the German Society of Anaesthesiology and Intensive Care Medicine and the Professional Association of German Anaesthetists. *Anaesth Intensivmed* 1989; **30**: 307–14.

48 Whitcher C, Ream AK, Parsons D *et al*. Anesthetic mishaps and the cost of monitoring: a proposed standard for monitoring equipment. *J Clin Monit* 1988; **4**: 5–15.

49 Winter A, Spence AA. Editorial. An international consensus on monitoring? *Br J Anaesth* 1990; **64**: 263–6.

50 Hamilton WK. Do we monitor enough? We monitor too much. *J Clin Monit* 1986; **2**: 264–6.

51 Hanning CD. Monitoring – bane or blessing? *Br J Anaesth* 1987; **59**: 1201–2.

52 Moyers J. Does monitoring have an effect on patient safety? Monitoring instruments are no substitute for careful clinical observation. *J Clin Monit* 1988; **4**: 107–11.

53 Cooper JB, Newbower RS, Kitz R. An analysis of major errors and equipment failures in anesthesia management: considerations for prevention and detection. *Anesthesiology* 1984; **60**: 34–42.

54 Cooper JB, Long CD, Newbower RS. Human error in anesthesia management. In: Grundy BL, Gravenstein JS, eds. *Quality of care in anesthesia*. Springfield: Charles C Thomas, 1982.

55 Chopra V, Bovill JG, Spierdijk J. Accidents, near accidents, and complications during anesthesia. *Anesthesiology* 1990; **45**: 3–6.

56 Denisco RA, Drummond JA, Gravenstein JS. The effect of fatigue on the performance of a simulated anesthetic monitoring task. *J Clin Monit* 1987; **3**: 22–4.

57 Johnson LC. Managing sleep to avoid fatigue. *Anaesth Educ* 1988; **5**: 13.

58 Parker J. The effects of fatigue on physician performance: an under-estimated cause of physician impairment and increased patient risk. *Can J Anaesth* 1987; **34**: 75–85.

59 Jackson SH. Humanism and anesthesia safety. *Curr Rev Clin Anaesth* 1988; **25** (8).

60 Harrison GG. Anaesthetic accidents. *Clin Anesth* 1983; **1**: 415–29.

61 Cooper JB, Newbower RS, Long CD, McPeek B. Preventable anesthetic mishaps – a study of human factors. *Anesthesiology* 1979; **49**: 339–406.

62 Cheney FW, Posner K, Caplan RA, Ward RJ. Standards of care and anesthesia liability. *JAMA* 1989; **261**: 1599–603.

63 Eichhorn JH. Prevention of intraoperative anesthesia accidents and related severe injury through safety monitoring. *Anesthesiology* 1989; **70**: 572–7.

64 Tinker JH, Dull DL, Caplan RA, Ward RJ, Cheney FW. Role of monitoring devices in prevention of anesthetic mishaps: a closed claims analysis. *Anesthesiology* 1989; **71**: 541–6.

65 Scott CD. Stress management can lead to reduced malpractice. *Phys Executive* 1988; **14**: 18–20.

66 Emmett C, Hutton P. Patient monitoring. *Br Med Bull* 1988; **44**: 302–21.

67 Petty C. Monitoring development in the USA. In: Hutton P, Prys-Roberts C eds. *Monitoring in anaesthesia and intensive care.* London: WB Saunders Co, 1994.

68 Orkin FK. Practice standards: the Midas touch or the Emperor's new clothes. *Anesthesiology* 1989; **70**: 567–71.

69 European Standard EN 475 – *Medical devices – electrically generated alarm signals.* Brussels: Committée Européan de Normalisation (CEN), 1995

70 International Standards Organisation (ISO) Standard ISO 9703. *Part 1: Visual alarm signals.* Geneva: International Standards Organisation, 1992. (Note: The corresponding British Standard, BS 7618: Part 1: 1992, was withdrawn on publication of EN 475: 1995)

71 International Standards Organisation (ISO) Standard ISO 9703. *Part 2: Auditory alarm signals.* Geneva: International Standards Organisation, 1994.

72 ASTM. *Specification for alarm signals in medical equipment used in anesthesia and respiratory care (F1463–93).* Philadelphia: American Society for Testing and Materials (ASTM), 1993.

73 Griffith RL, Raciot BM. A survey of practising anesthesiologists on auditory alarms in the operating room. In: Hedley-Whyte J, ed. *Operating room and intensive care alarms and information transfer (STP 1152).* Philadelphia: American Society for Testing and Materials (ASTM), 1992: 10–18.

74 Veitergribes J. Doucek C, Smith W. *Aircraft alerting systems criteria study (Report FAA Rd-76–222, 1 and 2).* Washington, DC: Federal Aviation Authority, 1977.

75 Sorkin RD, Woods DD. Systems with human monitors. A signal detection analysis. *Hum Computer Interaction* 1985; **1**: 49–75.

76 Patterson RD. Guidelines for the design of auditory warning sounds. *Proc Inst Accoustics* 1989; **11**: 17–25.

77 Patterson RD. Auditory warning sounds in the work environment. *Phil Trans R Soc Lond* 1990; **B327**: 485–92.

78 Patterson R. *Guidelines for auditory warning systems on civil aircraft.* London: Civil Aviation Authority Report No 82017, 1982.

79 Edworthy J, Loxley S, Dennis I. Improving auditory warning design: Relationship between warning sound parameters and perceived urgency. *Hum Factors* 1991; **33**: 205–231.

80 Meredith C, Edworthy J. Are there too many alarms in the intensive care unit? An overview of the problems. *J Adv Nurs* 1995; **21**: 15–20.

81 Westenskow DR. Alarms. In: Saidman LJ, Smith NT. *Monitoring in anesthesia.* Boston: Butterworth-Heinemann, 1993: 486.

82 Jones D, Lawson A, Holland R. Integrated monitor alarms and "alarm overload". *Anaesth Intens Care* 1991; **19**: 101–2.

83 Wallace M, Ashman M. Volume and frequency of anesthetic alarms: are the current alarm systems appropriate for normal human ear aging? *J Clin Monit* 1991; 7: 134.

84 Finley GA, Cohen AJ. Perceived urgency and the anaesthetist: responses to common operating room monitor alarms. *Can J Anaesth* 1992; **38**: 958–64. (Note erratum in *Can J Anaesth* 1991; **39**: 102.)

85 Loeb RG, Jones BR, Lenard RA, Behrman K. Recognition accuracy of current operating room alarms. *Anesth Analg* 1992; **75**: 499–505.

86 Weinger MB. Proposed new sounds may make a bad situation worse. *Anesthesiology* 1991; **74**: 791–2.

87 Stanford LM, McIntyre JWR, Hogan. Audible alarm signals for anaesthesia monitorig equipment. *Int J Clin Monit Comput* 1985; **1**: 251–6.

88 Schreiber P, Schreiber J. Diagnosis and prevention of operator error and equipment failure. *Sem Anesth* 1989; **8**: 141–8.

89 Weingarten M. Prioritization of monitors for the detection of mishaps. *Sem Anesth* 1989; **8**: 1–12.

90 Keats AS. Anesthesia mortality in perspective. *Anesth Analg* 1990; **71**: 113–19.

91 Beneken JEW, Gravenstein JS. Sophisticated alarms in patient monitoring; a methodology based on systems engineering concepts. In: Gravenstein JS, Newbower RS, Ream AK, eds. *The automated anesthesia record and alarm systems.* Boston: Butterworth-Heinemann, 1987: 211–28.

92 Watt RC, Miller KE, Navabi MJ, Hameroff SR, Mylrea KC. An approach to "smart alarms" in anesthesia monitoring. *Anesthesiology* 1988; **69**: A241.

93 Pan PH, James CF. Effects of default alarm settings on alarm distribution in telemetric probe oximetry network in ward setting. *Anesthesiology* 1991; **75**: A405.

94 Hyman WA. Evaluation of alarm systems for medical equipment. *J Clin Eng* 1982; **7**: 223–7.

95 Spraker TE. Alarm strategies for anesthesia: where we've been; where we are now; and where we're going. *J Clin Monit* 1989; **5**: 301.

96 Blum LR. Equipment design and human limitation. *Anesthesiology* 1971; **35**: 101–2.

97 Dorsch JA, Dorsch SE. *Understanding anesthesia equipment*, 3rd edn. Baltimore: Williams and Wilkins, 1994: 689.

98 Nickalls RWD, Ramasubramanian R. *Interfacing the IBM-PC to medical equipment. The art of serial communication.* Cambridge: Cambridge University Press, 1995.

99 Fiegler A, Stead S. The medical information bus. *Biomed Instrum Technol* 1990; **24**: 101–11.

100 Dorsch JA, Dorsch SE. *Understanding anesthesia equipment*, 3rd edn. Baltimore: Williams and Wilkins, 1994: 688.

101 Westenskow DR, Loeb RG, Brunner JX, Pace NL. Expert alarms and autopilot in an anesthesia workstation. *Anesthesiology* 1988; **69**: A731.

102 Egbert TP, Westenskow DR. Detection of artifact in pulse oximetry signals using a neural network. *Anesthesiology* 1992; **77**: A521.

103 Fukui Y. An expert alarm system. In: Gravenstein J, Newbower R, Ream AK *et al. The automated anesthesia and alarm systems.* Stoneham, Mass: Butterworth, 1987: 203–9.

104 van der Aa JJ. *Intelligent alarms in anesthesia.* PhD dissertation, Eindhoven University, Netherlands, 1990.

105 Westenskow DR, Orr JA, Simon FH, Bender HJ, Frankenberger H. Intelligent alarms to reduce anesthesiologist's response time to critical faults. *Anesthesiology* 1992; **77**: 1074–9.

106 Watt RC, Navabi M, Mylrea K, Hameroff SR. Integrated monitoring "smart alarms" can detect critical events and reduce false alarms. *Anesthesiology* 1989; **71**: A338.

107 Philip JH. Overview: creating practical alarms for the future. *J Clin Monit* 1989; **5**: 194–5.

108 Goldman GH, Waterson CK, Lucas WJ. Smart anesthesia monitoring system: rule-based intubation detection. *IEEE Engineering in Medicine and Biology Society, 10th Annual Conference*, 1988.

109 Kalli S, Stapinovits J. Model based approach in intelligent patient monitoring. *IEEE Engineering in Medicine and Biology Society, 10th International Conference*, 1988.

110 Philip JH. Thoughtful alarms. In: Gravenstein JS, Newbower RS, Ream AK, eds. *The automated anesthesia record and alarm systems.* Boston: Butterworth-Heinemann, 1987.

111 Rennels GD, Miller PL. Artificial intelligence research in anesthesia and intensive care. *J Clin Monit* 1988; **4**: 274–89.
112 Loeb RG, Brunner JX, Westenskow DR, Feldman B, Pace NL. The Utah anesthesia workstation. *Anesthesiology* 1989; **70**: 999–1007.
113 Mylrea KC, Orr JA, Westenskow DR. Integration of monitoring for intelligent alarms in anesthesia: neural networks – can they help? *J Clin Monit* 1993; **9**: 31–7.
114 Fukui Y, Masuzawa T. Knowledge-based approach to intelligent alarms. *J Clin Monit* 1989; **5**: 211–16.
115 Mintz R, Ford D, Kaczorowski D. On-line identification and analysis of hemodynamic trends and patterns by use of rule-based knowledge representation. *Anesthesiology* 1987; **67**: 3A.

Bibliography

Blitt CM. *Monitoring in anesthesia and critical care medicine*, 2nd edn. London: Churchill-Livingstone, 1990.

Daily EK, Schroeder JS. *Techniques in bedside hemodynamic monitoring*, 5th edn. St. Louis: Mosby-Year Book, 1994.

Darovic, GO. *Hemodynamic monitoring: invasive and non-invasive clinical application*. Philadelphia: WB Saunders Company, 1987.

Davey A, Moyle JBT, Ward CS. *Ward's anaesthetic equipment*, 3rd edn. London: WB Saunders Company, 1992.

Ehrenwerth J, Eisenkraft JB. *Anesthesia equipment*. St. Louis: Mosby-Year Book, 1993.

Geddes LA. *The direct and indirect measurement of blood pressure*. Chicago, Year Book Publishers Inc, 1970.

Geddes LA. *Cardiovascular devices and their applications*. New York: John Wiley & Sons, 1984.

Geddes LA, Baker LE. *Principles of applied biomedical instrumentation*, 3rd edn. New York: John Wiley & Sons, 1989.

Gravenstein JS, Paulus, DA. *Clinical monitoring practice*, 2nd edn. Philadelphia: JB Lippincott Company, 1987.

Hutton P, Prys-Roberts, C. *Monitoring in anaesthesia and intensive care*. London: WB Saunders Company Ltd, 1994.

Lake CL. *Clinical monitoring*, 2nd edn. Philadelphia: WB Saunders Company, 1995.

Mathie RT, ed. *Blood flow measurement in man*. Tunbridge Wells, Kent: Castle House Publications, 1982.

Prys-Roberts C. Measurement of cardiac output and regional blood flow. In Prys-Roberts, C. ed. *The circulation in anaesthesia*. Oxford: Blackwell Scientific Publicactions, 1980.

Saidman LJ, Smith NT. *Monitoring in anaesthesia*, 3rd edn. Boston: Butterworth-Heinemann, 1993.

Smith NT. Non-invasive assessment of the cardiovascular system. In Prys-Roberts, C. ed. *The circulation in anaesthesia*, Oxford: Blackwell Scientific publications, 1980.

Swales JD ed. *Textbook of hypertension*. Oxford: Blackwell Scientific, 1995.

Sykes MK, Vickers MD, Hull CJ. *Principles of measurement and monitoring in anaesthesia and intensive care*, 3rd edn. Oxford: Blackwell Scientific Publications, 1991.

Taylor KJW, Burns PN, Wells PN (eds). *Clinical applications of Doppler ultrasound*. London: Academic Press, 1988.

Thys DM, Kaplan JA. *The ECG in anesthesia and critical care*. New York: Churchill Livingstone, 1987.

Waeber B, O'Brien E, O'Malley K, Brunner HR eds. *Ambulatory blood pressure*. New York: Raven Press, 1994.

Figure references

A Hutton P, Prys-Roberts C, eds. *Monitoring in Anaesthesia and Intensive Care*. London, WB Saunders Company Ltd, 1994.

B Saidman LJ, Smith NT, eds. *Monitoring in anesthesia*, 3rd ed. Boston, Butterworth Heinemann, 1993.

C Sykes MK, Vickers MD, Hull CJ. *Principles of measurement and monitoring in anaesthesia and intensive care*, 3rd ed. Oxford, Blackwell, 1991.

D Davey A, Moyle JBT, Ward CS. *Ward's Anaesthetic Equipment*, 3rd ed. London, WB Saunders Company Ltd, 1992.

E Darovic GO. *Hemodynamic monitoring*. Philadelphia, WB Saunders Company, 1989.

F Blitt CD, Hines RL, eds. *Monitoring in anesthesia and critical care medicine*, 3rd ed. New York, Church Livingstone, 1995.

Other sources are cited against the diagrams concerned.

Index

myocardial infarction 45
myocardial ischaemia 42–3, 171, 173
myocardial wall motion 173

negligence, medical 4–5
neonatal medicine
    alarms 200, 210
    Doppler ultrasound monitoring 169
    thoracic impedance monitoring 193
nerve damage 99, 146
noise
    pollution 200, 208
    rejection, ECG machines 15–17
non-invasive cardiovascular monitoring
    1–2
    clinical application 3–4
    cost implications 6
    historical outline 3
    medico-legal aspects 4–5
    merits 2
    methodologies 6–7
nurses
    alarms and 209, 210–11
    blood pressure monitoring 126–9
    community see community nurses
    ECG monitoring 43–4, 46–7
    ultrasound monitoring 178
Nyquist limit 167

obesity, sphygmomanometry in 73, 76,
    79
observer error, blood pressure
    measurement 112–13
obstetrics
    blood pressure monitoring 106, 125,
    144
    thoracic impedance cardiography
    193
oesophageal ECG leads 20, 21
Ohm's law 23
oscillometry 64, 82–4
    abandonment/rediscovery 84
    automated see automated blood
    pressure monitors
    practical applications 90–1, 127
    sources of error 114, 117
oscillotonometry 64, 82, 84–90
    automated see automated blood
    pressure monitors
    popularity and limitations 90
    potential problems 89–90
    practical applications 90–1, 127
    sources of error 90, 114, 115, 117

paediatrics
    ambulatory blood pressure
    monitoring 133
    blood pressure monitoring 62–3,
    64–5, 99, 122
    Doppler ultrasound monitoring 169
    normal blood pressure values 61
    thoracic impedance monitoring 191,
    193
palpation 61–2, 122, 152
parallax errors 113
paramedical personnel, blood pressure
    monitoring 129–30
Penaz "unloaded artery" principle 104,
    105
phaeochromocytoma 133
pharmacists, blood pressure
    monitoring 130
phase distortion, ECG waveform 31,
    32
physical constraints,
    sphygmomanometry 79
physiotherapists 129
piezo-electric effect 163
pitch 159–60
plethysmography
    in blood pressure monitoring 63–4,
    105–8
    impedance 186
    in pulse monitoring 153
    sources of error 115
pleural effusion 193
Poiseuille's manometer 53, 54
Portapres 107
positive end-expiratory pressure
    (PEEP) 167, 174, 191
posture
    blood pressure and 60
    sphygmomanometry 71, 78–9
potentials
    electrode 18
    electrode–skin 23
power, ultrasound 163
pre-eclampsia 125, 146, 193
pregnancy, blood pressure monitoring
    125, 144
P–R interval 27
protocols, home blood pressure
    monitoring 147
pulmonary oedema 190, 193
pulse 6
    monitoring 152–6
    conditions for 154
    problems 155
    monitors 65, 152–4
    palpation 61–2, 122, 152

detection methods 163–4
diagnostic scope and limitations 176–8
Doppler *see* Doppler ultrasound
hazards 164
theory/physics 158–64
U-wave 28

varicose veins 175
vascular surgery 176, 179
Vasotrac tonometer system 108
veins, varicose 175
velocity
Doppler measurement 160–1, 162

sound 158–9, 160
velography, aortic 165–9, 178
venous occlusion 165, 176, 178
venous thrombosis, deep 165, 175–6, 179
Vierordt's sphygmograph 53
von Recklinghausen, H 54, 82, 84, 86

wall motion, myocardial 173
wavelength, sound 158–9, 160
"white coat" hypertension 112, 122, 134

zero errors, blood pressure measurement 113–14